HIGH-PERFORMANCE
BODYBUILDING

HIGH-PERFORMANCE
BODYBUILDING

John Parrillo
and Maggie Greenwood-Robinson

Foreword by Robert Kennedy
Publisher of *MuscleMag International*

A Perigee Book

Individual dietary needs vary, and no one diet will meet everyone's requirements. Before beginning any diet or exercise program, consult your physician. Do not take nutritional supplements without your physician's approval. Responsibility for any adverse effects or unforeseen consequences resulting from the use of the information contained herein is expressly disclaimed.

Perigee Books
are published by
The Putnam Publishing Group
200 Madison Avenue
New York, NY 10016

Library of Congress Cataloging-in-Publication Data

Parrillo, John.
    High-performance bodybuilding / by John Parrillo and Maggie
Greenwood-Robinson ; foreword by Robert Kennedy.
        p.   cm.
    ''A Perigee book.''
    ISBN 0-399-51771-5 (alk. paper)
    1. Bodybuilding. 2. Nutrition. 3. Diet. I. Greenwood-Robinson,
Maggie. II. Title.
GV546.5.P38   1993   92-15571 CIP
646.7'5—dc20

Cover design by Andrew M. Newman
Cover photo © 1992 by Image Source
Cover model: Dave Hawk
Exercise models: Bob Cicherillo, Dennis Newman, Lisa Lorio, and Jana Holmes
Exercise and fascial stretch photography: Jimmie D. King
Photograph of John Parrillo by Barry Brooks
Printed in the United States of America
1 2 3 4 5 6 7 8 9 10

This book is printed on acid-free paper.

To Nicole

Contents

Acknowledgments

This book has become a reality, thanks to the efforts of many people:

Maggie Greenwood-Robinson, my co-author, who had the idea to do the book and was a driving force behind it;

Robert Kennedy, who believed in the project from its inception and graciously promoted it for us;

Greg Zulak, who brought my nutrition and training programs to the attention of the world with his well-crafted articles in *MuscleMag International* and *FLEX*;

Lou Zwick, producer of "American Muscle" on ESPN, who has been generous in featuring Parrillo Performance on his popular show;

Joe Weider, the late Bill Reynolds, and the editorial staff of *FLEX* who were good enough to run a comprehensive series of articles on my programs in their magazine;

My staff at Parrillo Performance, who provide guidance each day to the hundreds of bodybuilders and athletes who call our offices;

Jimmie D. King, who photographed the exercises and fascial stretches; Barry Brooks, who assisted; as well as the other photographers who provided photos: J. M. Manion, Jim Amentler, and Paul B. Goode.

Cliff Sheats, certified clinical nutritionist and colleague, who has been a constant source of support and information;

Eugene Brissie, our publisher, who recognized the possibilities in this book;

And most importantly, all the hard-training bodybuilders, who have made my work possible. These are people who, through dedication to proper nutrition and training, believed they could achieve new levels of excellence—and did.

John Parrillo
Cincinnati, Ohio

Foreword

The name John Parrillo is magic in body-building circles. In all my years in this sport, rarely have I met a person whose nutrition and training techniques were so innovative—and so dramatically effective. It seems that no matter what major contest I attend, I learn that the top three or four competitors are disciples of John Parrillo and his methods. Many top bodybuilders who are near or at their genetic limits have made remarkable gains by following John's programs.

In 1990, my magazine, *MuscleMag International,* ran a lengthy article on John Parrillo by Greg Zulak, who called his subject a "genius who knows more about losing body fat and maximizing muscle than anyone." The more I learned about John's programs, the more I could understand Greg's enthusiasm. Here was a man who had bodybuilders eating up to 10,000 calories a day and maintaining body-fat levels of below 10 percent! What was he doing to get these kind of results?

I have concluded that John Parrillo has created the most comprehensive—and groundbreaking—approach to bodybuild-ing I have ever seen. Diet, supplements, medium-chain triglycerides, training, aerobics, stretching—these are the elements, cohesively working together to help people lose fat and gain muscle. It is underpinned by this astounding philosophy of eating more calories.

I want any bodybuilder, athlete, or exerciser who has not already heard of John Parrillo to try his programs. They are different. They are grounded in nutritional science. Most of all, they help you get what all bodybuilders want: lean mass. I think that once you commit yourself to John's methods, you'll not turn back. He has created a bodybuilding system you'll stick to for life.

It has been a long time since the sport of bodybuilding has witnessed anything that can be described as truly revolutionary. At long last we have John Parrillo, who has, without question, revolutionized the way we diet and train.

Robert Kennedy
Publisher, *MuscleMag International*

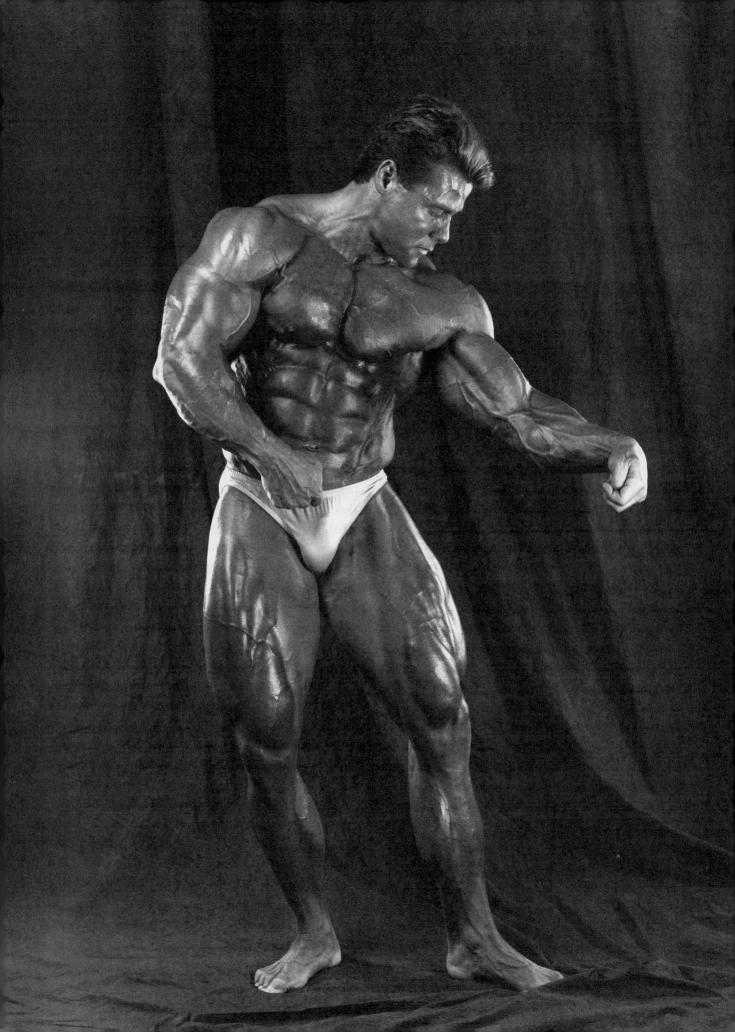

ONE

BODYBUILDING BREAKTHROUGHS

A major transformation in your physique is about to take place. Once and for all, you can get leaner and more muscular than you ever thought possible. You can have more energy than you ever dreamed. You can start feeling better about yourself than you have in years. And, you can do it all by following some truly breakthrough bodybuilding techniques that will help you achieve the best shape of your life.

First, I'll introduce you to a high-calorie nutrition program that burns fat and builds muscle. If you're like most bodybuilders, you've probably tried to lose body fat by drastically cutting calories on all sorts of diets, from low-carbohydrate regimens to gimmicky food plans. Fad diets like these never work as well as you want them to. Instead of losing just body fat, you lose a lot of hard-earned muscle in the process.

The solution to losing body fat—and keeping it off—will totally amaze you. The solution to losing body fat lies not in cutting calories, but in increasing them.

It's true. As remarkable as this sounds, you can burn fat on a high-calorie diet—

Dave Hawk has the right package of mass and muscularity. Photo by J. M. Manion.

and build muscle at the same time.

Next, I'll tell you about my nutritional supplementation program, which includes the use of medium-chain fatty acid (MCFA) oil, a natural supplement with some remarkable applications in sports nutrition, as well as several other important bodybuilding supplements. With supplements included in the diet, your digestive system processes more nutrients. In turn, the nutrient levels in your body increase at the cellular level—beyond what can be achieved by food alone—and this stimulates metabolic processes for fat-burning and muscle-building.

From there, I'll show you how to use nutrition and supplementation to gain muscle mass. This topic should be of special interest to competitive bodybuilders and other athletes who want to pack on as much muscle as possible in the off-season.

Then, I'll go into the specifics of how you can put your body into a fat-burning mode on a 12-week, three-stage fat-loss program. It's designed for competitive bodybuilders who are preparing for contests and for noncompetitive bodybuilders and athletes who want to reduce their body-fat levels. This fat-loss program

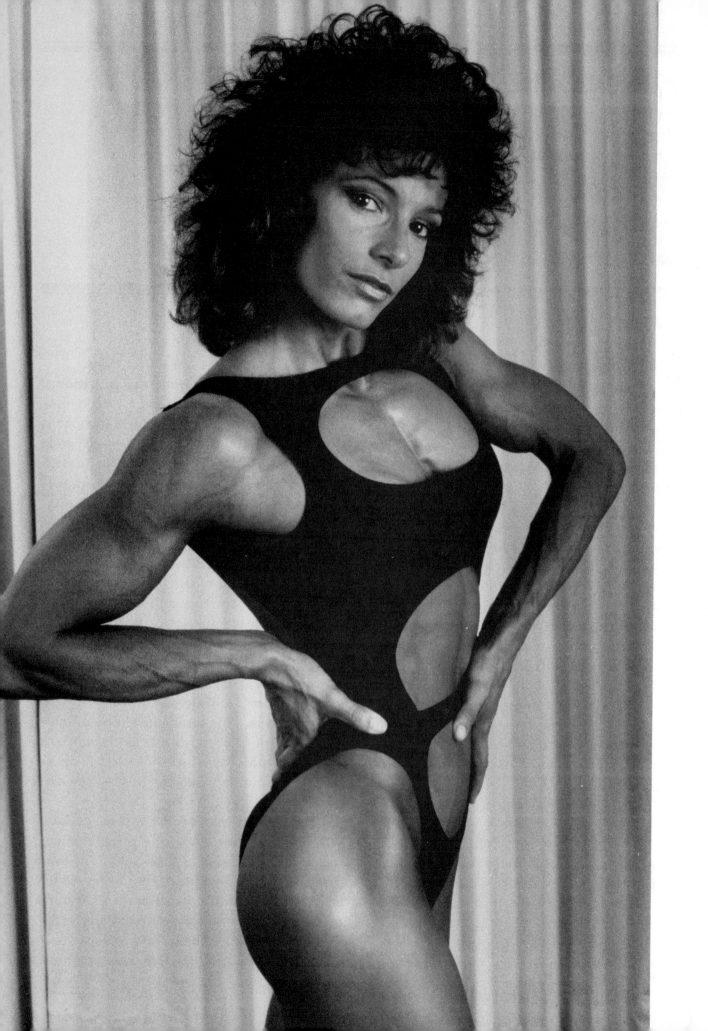

helps you get lean, stay muscular, and have plenty of energy to train hard.

Finally, I'll explain my training techniques. Some are rather basic, while others are quite revolutionary. Take my fascial stretching, for example. This is a special training technique I developed so that bodybuilders and athletes can develop greater muscular size, shape, and separation.

All of these nutrition and training techniques are designed to work together. Followed with 100 percent commitment, these techniques get results, regardless of whether you train for competition, for fitness, or for both.

CASE STUDIES

From Cincinnati, Ohio, where my business, Parrillo Performance, is located, I work with bodybuilders and athletes from all over the world, advising them on how to develop lean muscle mass through proper nutrition and training. To many bodybuilders and athletes, the goal of gaining muscle while staying lean seems out of reach. But once they try my techniques for themselves, they discover just how attainable their goals really are. Here are a few case studies:

A high body-fat percentage was a problem for one top female bodybuilder, even though she had a very symmetrical physique. Attempting to lose her fat, she was eating roughly 1,000 calories a day. I explained to her that this severe restriction in calories was making her metabolism so sluggish that she could not possibly burn fat. I increased her calories to 4,000 a

day and advised her on the proper foods and nutritional supplements to include in that caloric allotment. Fueled by improved nutrition, she increased her aerobics to three times a day, adopted my exercise techniques, and began to work out with a new level of intensity.

At the end of 10 days, I measured her body-fat-to-lean-muscle ratio. As amazing as it seems, she had lost 10 pounds of body fat and gained four pounds of muscle. She was running an easy five miles a day, where once she could barely go 50 yards. In just over a week, she had achieved her best shape and conditioning ever.

Another top-ranked bodybuilder came to me because he needed more size to be competitive. At 5′ 8″ tall, he weighed 194 pounds. His goal was to increase his weight to 225 pounds, but I knew he could go much higher. After working with him for only four months, I helped him reach a body weight of more than 240 pounds. Incredibly, his body fat stayed the same as it was when he weighed 194. In other words, his gain was pure muscle! And, he did it by eating 9,800 calories a day, incorporating fascial stretching in his workouts, following my weight-training techniques, and doing aerobics for an hour every day.

One rather skinny bodybuilder consulted me because he had never been able to achieve the size he wanted, despite years of training and trying every nutritional supplement on the market. I told him to forget about supplements for the time being and to concentrate on proper nutrition. He followed my recommendations to the letter, and for the first time ever, steadily gained muscle mass. By the end of six months, this bodybuilder had gained 50 pounds, and not an ounce of it was fat.

Besides being a popular pro bodybuilder, Penny Price is a top fitness model. Photo by Jimmie D. King.

Not too long ago I received an inspiring letter from an up-and-coming body-builder. A year before, he was involved in a near-fatal motorcycle accident, which incapacitated him for seven weeks. His doctor thought he would permanently lose full range of movement on his right side.

Still on crutches, this young man returned to the gym and started doing as much work as he could, and at the same time, he began my nutrition and training programs. Months later, he won the Light Heavyweight Class at the Continental USA with better shape, size, and muscular definition than he had ever shown before in competition. The judges were amazed at the progress he had made in one year. Then he told them about the accident, and they were astounded. His amazing—and speedy—recovery has convinced him of the importance of nutrients in the healing process.

Competitive bodybuilders are not the only ones who benefit from my programs. If you train with weights as part of your fitness program, you can make much faster progress if you follow the nutrition and training recommendations outlined in this book. Case in point: A machinist came to me because he had always wanted to look more muscular—not like a bodybuilder but more like a well-trained athlete. When he first started working with me, he was thin and wiry, with very poor, slumped-over posture. He started my diet and began working out using my training methods, including fascial stretching. Just two months later, he had transformed his physique by gaining 15 pounds of muscle, while significantly reducing his body fat. In addition, his posture had improved enormously.

In another case, a noncompetitive bodybuilder who weight-trained reli-giously for 20 years had to stop working out for a full year, following surgery to repair detached retinas in both eyes. As soon as his doctor said he could resume training, he did—and started my nutrition program at the same time. In just 12 weeks, he gained 10 pounds of muscle and added more size to his frame than he had been able to do in all his prior years of training. As a self-professed "hard gai-ner," he was amazed by his progress, particularly because of his age (47).

Speaking of age, in 1992 I published the testimonial of a 78-year-old man in my newsletter, *The Parrillo Performance Press.* This fellow wrote that early in his life, he trained with weights but always inconsistently. Not only that, he had very poor eating habits. Some years ago, he started my nutrition program and stayed on it, along with training regularly three days a week. He was able to gain more muscle than he ever had before. From the picture he sent me, he looks about 20 years younger than he actually is.

Many personal trainers around the country are sanctioned to use my nutrition and training programs with their clients. A trainer from the Northeast told me recently about one of his students, a 39-year-old woman who was overweight and wanted to get in better shape. The trainer put her on my nutrition program, and she lost 30 pounds over the course of a few months. When the pounds came off, the trainer noticed that this woman had potential as a competitive bodybuilder. After some initial persuasion, she began training for her first bodybuilding competition.

My nutrition and training programs also work for endurance athletes by making them leaner, stronger, and thus faster. A good example is a pro triathlete from New Jersey, who dropped his body fat levels

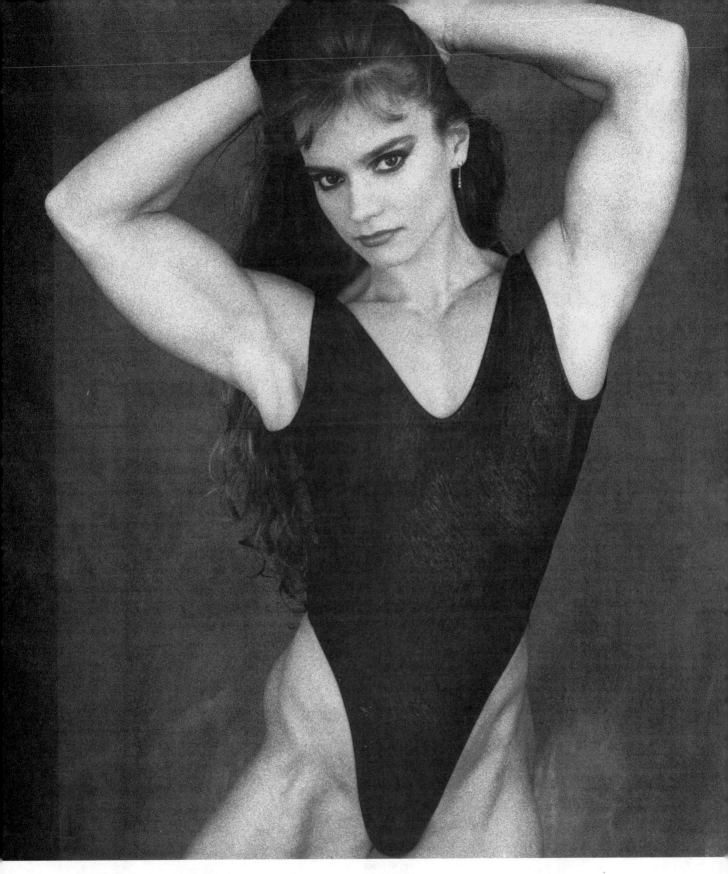

Julia Kover is a favorite on the bodybuilding scene.
Photo by Paul B. Goode.

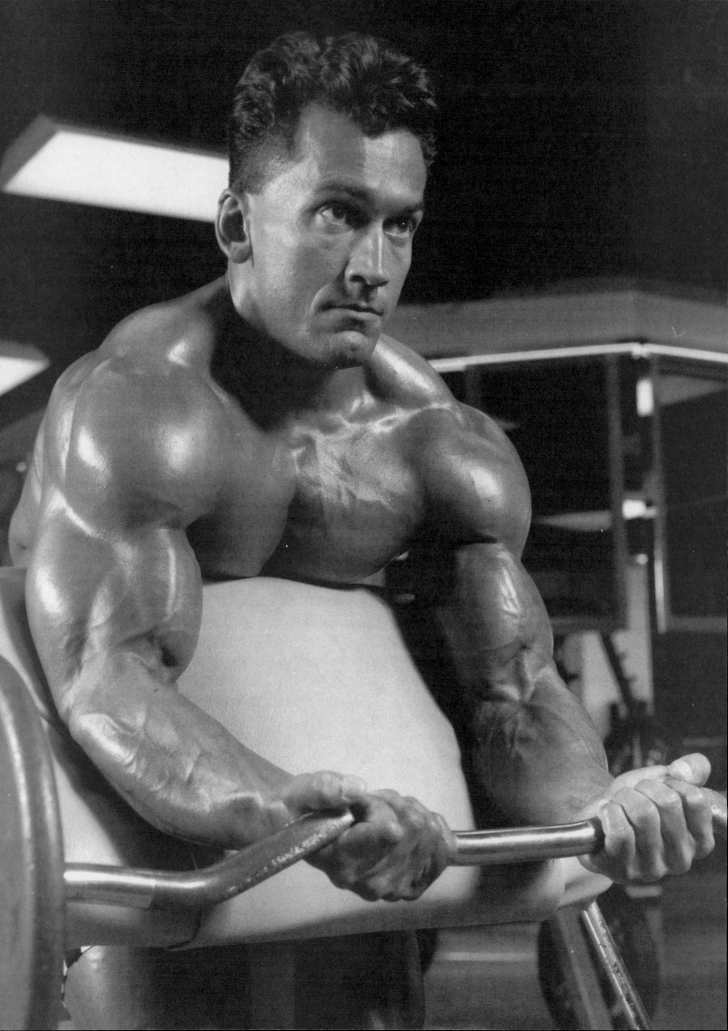

significantly—all by eating 6,000 calories a day. In a qualifier race for his third Iron-man, the toughest, most grueling triath-lon in the world, he was able to maintain a sub-six-minute pace and turned in the third-fastest race of the day.

Once in the Ironman, he was fueled by a breakfast of egg whites and oatmeal. During the first half of the bike race, he consumed 32 ounces of a special carbo-hydrate drink, mixed with a medium-chain fatty acid supplement. He dismounted his bicycle in 240th place (out of 1,450 professional competitors). At the 19th-mile marker, he had moved up to 110th place. With seven miles to go, he picked up his pace and finished in 79th place—his strongest Ironman showing ever.

These are just a few examples of the many successes bodybuilders and ath-letes throughout the country have experi-enced with my nutrition and training programs. These athletes are learning how to reduce body-fat levels and build muscle faster and more efficiently than ever—all while maintaining plenty of en-ergy and stamina for rigorous training.

The results are dramatic, even remark-able. Most importantly, they are possible. By applying some very easy-to-follow techniques in nutrition, supplementation, and training—and doing it with consist-ency and dedication—you can achieve the results you want. It all begins with proper nutrition.

A 100 percent commitment to nutrition is what makes champions such as Lee Labrada. Photo by Jim Amentler.

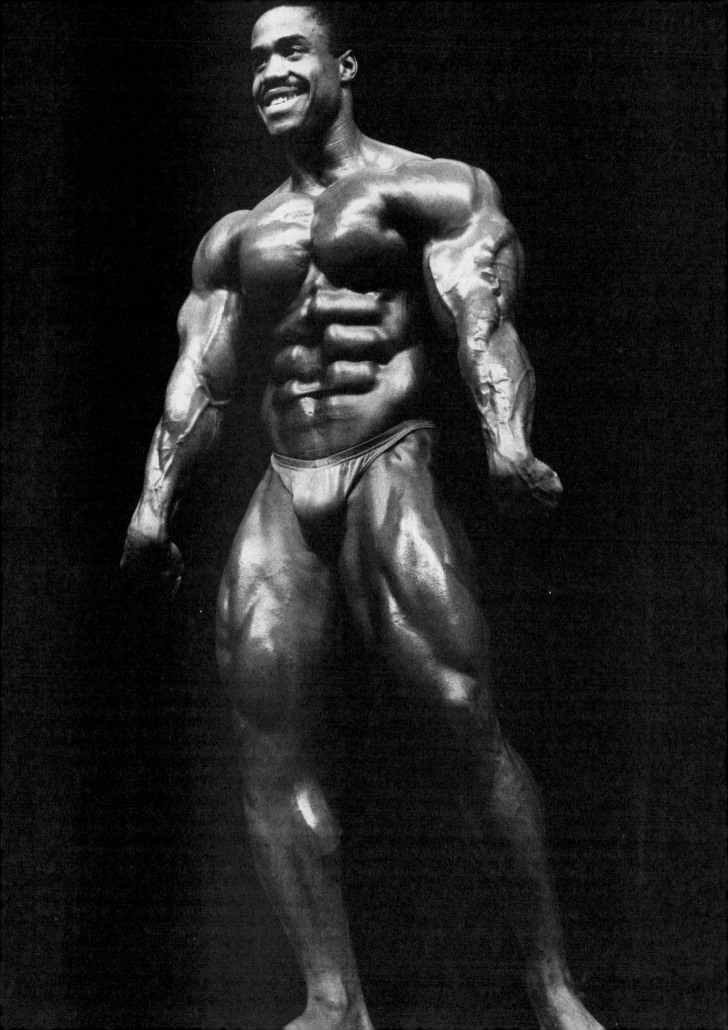

TWO
A SCIENTIFIC APPROACH TO BUILDING LEAN MASS

I learned the importance of proper nutrition during my days as a competitive bodybuilder, but I learned it the hard way. The first bodybuilding diet I ever followed was a zero-carbohydrate regimen. For six weeks, I subsisted on nothing but cherry-flavored liquid protein. Before long, I was feeling faint and dizzy. Worse yet, I was losing all the muscle I worked so hard to build. Realizing that there must be a better way to get lean and stay muscular, I began a lifelong study of nutrition that included intensive research in the physical and biological sciences. At the same time, I started working with top-level amateur and professional bodybuilders, helping them with their diets and training programs.

My research and work with bodybuilders led to the creation of a scientific-based nutrition program that "builds the metabolism" for optimum fat loss and muscular growth. Many popular diets claim to stimulate the metabolism. In reality, however, they are the same old low-calorie regimes but wrapped in new packages. Low-calorie diets like these are the least effective because they drastically cut caloric intake, resulting in muscle loss, body-fat retention, and low energy levels.

DIETARY CONTROL OF METABOLISM

You're probably familiar with this common dilemma among bodybuilders: how to gain muscle mass without getting fat. To a large extent, the solution to this dilemma involves dietary control of your metabolism—providing your body with the components it needs for synthesizing muscle, not body fat.

Metabolism is the breakdown and conversion of food to energy for growth and repair. It has two components: catabolism and anabolism. Catabolism is the dismantling of nutrients from food to provide energy and building blocks for growth. Anabolism is the construction of new body tissues from these nutrient building blocks. Simply put, anabolism means growth. This is why growth-pro-

The Natural Wonder Mike Ashley knows the value of proper nutrition. Photo by J. M. Manion.

ducing substances are said to be "anabolic"—because they stimulate growth. Your body produces its own such substances, and my nutrition program is designed to help you take maximum advantage of what your body can accomplish naturally.

FOOD FOR FUEL AND MUSCLE

During metabolism, three things can happen: 1) The food is burned to release energy; 2) It is broken down into nutrients to be used by the body for growth and repair; 3) Nutrients from the breakdown of food are excreted. Because your body is efficient at absorbing nutrients, very few are excreted without being used.

If you consume nutrients in excess of what is required to support your current weight and level of activity, the additional calories will be converted into more body weight, either muscle or body fat. My nutrition program is designed specifically to supply the building blocks your body needs to construct new muscle—not the building blocks to make fat.

There is a difference. The same number of calories from different foods has different effects on your body weight. This is very easy to prove. Just try replacing 1,000 calories of potatoes and brown rice

Dean Caputo (left) is an old friend from my powerlifting days. Photo by Jimmie D. King.

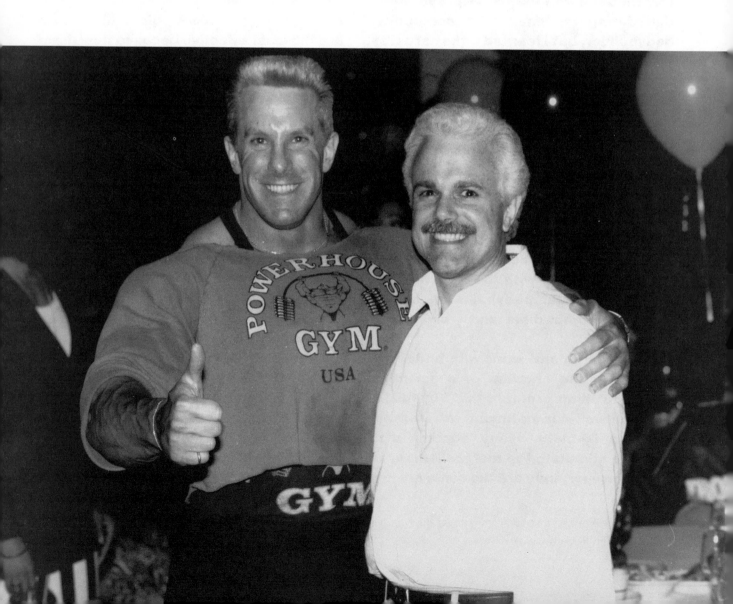

with 1,000 calories of candy and ice cream in your diet, and see what happens to your body-fat levels.

Conventional dietary fat and foods containing it (including fatty cuts of meat) tend to be easily stored as body fat. The reason is, the chemical composition of dietary fat is similar to that of body fat, and so very little energy is needed to turn dietary fat into body fat. By contrast, protein and carbohydrate must be chemically converted to fat before they can be stored as fat. The conversion process uses up a portion of the calories contained in the protein or carbohydrate food, and this expenditure reduces the tendency of these foods to be converted to body fat.

Simple sugars such as glucose, fructose, lactose, and sucrose are easily converted to body fat, although to a lesser extent than conventional fat. When simple sugars are released into the bloodstream faster than the body can use them to replenish glycogen stores or meet energy requirements, an overproduction of the hormone insulin occurs. This insulin response causes fat cells to take up the excess sugar and turn it into body fat. As you'll learn later in this book, insulin is important in the process of protein synthesis for muscle growth; yet, paradoxically, too much stimulates fat production.

METABOLISM-BUILDING NUTRITION

The ideal bodybuilding diet is one that builds the metabolism so that you can consume plenty of calories, lose body fat quickly, gain muscle, and have the energy to train with all-out intensity every workout. That's just what my nutrition program does. Here's how it works:

Increase Your Calories.

To lose body fat, most bodybuilders think they must severely restrict their caloric intake. But when denied food, the body begins to feed on the protein in the muscles. Because muscle is the body's most metabolically active tissue, depleting it interferes with your ability to burn calories. Plus, restrictive diets lower your metabolic rate, making it easier for your body to store fat.

On my nutrition program, you gradually increase calories to lose body fat and gain muscle. Depending on your sex, size, activity level, and present metabolic state, you eat between 2,000 calories a day and 10,000 a day, sometimes more.

Select Only Metabolism-building Foods.

When you're attempting to lose body fat and gain muscle, food selection becomes critical. To effectively build your metabolism for fat-burning and muscle-building, you must know exactly what kinds of foods to eat, what to avoid, and how to properly structure your meals. Here are foods you eat on my nutrition program:

Lean Protein. Protein has a number of functions in the body: It is involved in the growth, maintenance, and repair of cells; it helps create hemoglobin, which carries oxygen to cells; it is required for the formation of antibodies to ward off disease and infection; and it helps produce enzymes and hormones for the regulation of body processes.

Protein is made up of organic compounds called amino acids, which are required by every metabolic process. Your body needs 22 amino acids in a certain balance to synthesize protein for muscu-

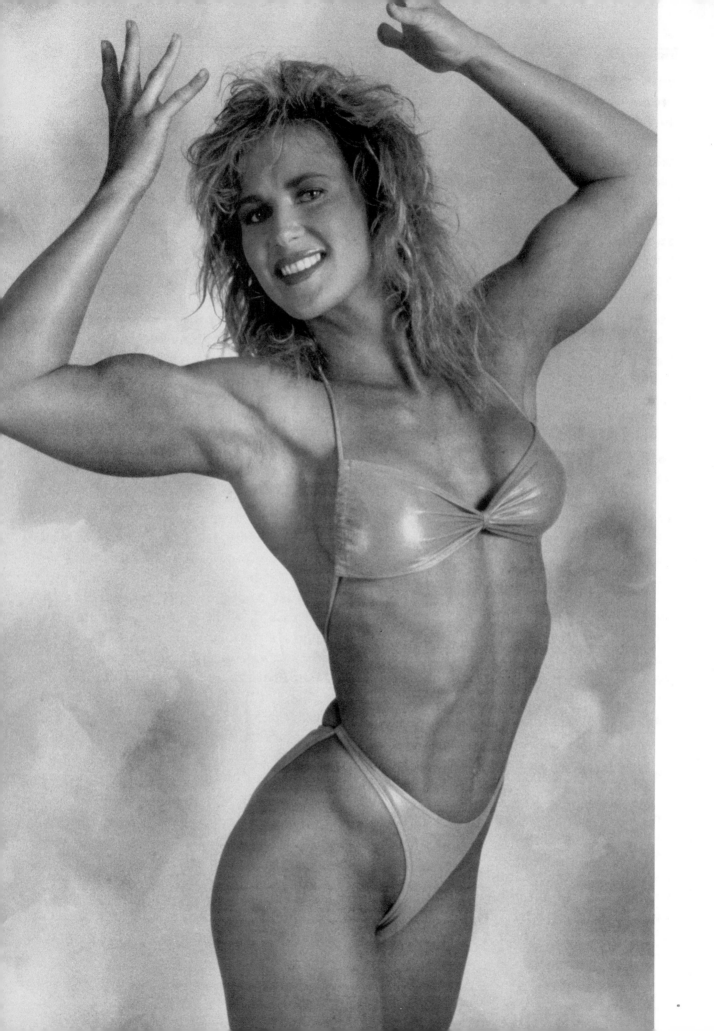

lar growth. All but eight of the amino acids can be manufactured by the body. Those eight are called "essential amino acids," and they are supplied by animal proteins such as chicken and fish. Foods that contain the eight essential amino acids are called "complete proteins."

Without enough protein in your diet, the body cannot properly support growth and repair or drive the metabolic processes. Bodybuilders have higher-than-normal requirements for protein because the muscles use more amino acids during training.

Of all foods, protein has the highest "dynamic action" on the metabolism. This describes the ability of a food to stimulate the body's metabolic rate. All foods do this to some extent. Studies, however, have shown that a high-protein meal raises the metabolic rate more than 30 percent in a 10-to-12-hour period, whereas carbohydrates and fats increase the metabolic rate approximately 4 percent over the same time period.

Most of your protein should come from complete, low-fat sources such as white-meat chicken and turkey, fish, and egg whites.

Carbohydrates. Next on your list of foods are carbohydrates, which provide the main source of energy for your body. During digestion, carbohydrates are broken down into glucose, also known as blood sugar, which is used as energy for the red blood cells and the central nervous system. Glucose is also the chief source of energy used by the muscles during exercise, particularly in the first ten minutes. When not used immediately by the body, glucose is stored in the liver and muscles as glycogen.

April Johnson knows how to keep her body fat levels low. Photo by Jimmie D. King.

Long, intense workouts can easily deplete glycogen stores. If the muscles cannot get enough glycogen, fatigue sets in, and endurance and performance drop considerably. A carbohydrate-rich diet prevents these side effects.

I divide carbohydrates into two categories: starchy and fibrous. Starchy carbohydrates have a high carbohydrate and calorie content and supply a slow, steady release of glucose—unlike simple sugars such as sugar or candy, which produce a sharp rise in blood sugar. In addition, the body stores a slightly higher percentage of glycogen from starchy carbohydrates than it does from simple sugars. Excellent sources of starchy carbohydrates include oatmeal, oat bran, any unrefined cereal, brown rice, potatoes, sweet potatoes, yams, corn, peas, lima beans, kidney beans, and all legumes.

As the name implies, fibrous carbohydrates are high in fiber, which is necessary for a healthy digestive tract. These carbohydrates are also lower in calories. Fibrous carbohydrates include broccoli, cauliflower, spinach, green beans, and all salad vegetables.

Essential Fats. Some dietary fat is essential for good health because it furnishes the body with nutrients called "essential fatty acids" or EFAs. Involved in many biological functions, EFAs are vital for normal growth, a healthy circulatory system, a healthy nervous system, and strong connective tissue and cell walls. EFAs also keep the skin healthy by enhancing elasticity and preventing dryness. Deficiencies in EFAs can cause poor skin tone and aching joints.

In my nutrition program, dietary fats should be kept as low as possible. You must, however, have EFAs in your diet. Each day, take one teaspoon to one tablespoon of an EFA source such as safflower, sunflower, linseed, or flaxseed oils.

Combine Foods Properly.

Each meal should be structured to include a lean protein, one or two starchy carbohydrates, and one or two fibrous carbohydrates. This combination of foods has two important benefits: First, the protein and fiber slow the digestion of carbohydrates—and consequently the release of glucose—to provide consistent energy levels and sustained endurance throughout the day. Second, this combination provides a constant supply of nutrients so that your body can maintain its energy, growth, and repair status.

Eat Five to Six Meals a Day or More, Spaced Two to Three Hours Apart.

This pattern of eating is metabolically beneficial—for three reasons. First, it helps naturally elevate your body's levels of insulin, a hormone with powerful anabolic (growth-producing) effects. One of its chief roles in the body is to make amino acids available to muscle tissue for growth and recovery. Insulin's release is triggered by the conversion of carbohydrate into glucose by the liver. When glucose is introduced into the bloodstream, the pancreas releases insulin in response.

For growth to occur, insulin must be constantly present in the body so that amino acids and glucose can move into muscle tissue. Following a meal, amino acids remain available for protein synthesis for only about three hours. By eating meals of protein and carbohydrate two to three hours apart, you ensure that your system is releasing adequate amounts of insulin, which, in turn, can exert its growth-producing action.

The second reason frequent meals are beneficial involves "thermogenesis"—the production of body heat from the burning of food for energy. Following a meal, your metabolic rate is elevated as a result of thermogenesis. Consequently, the more meals you eat, the higher your metabolic rate stays throughout the day.

Third, with a constant nutrient supply, you are never forced into a "starvation mode," a state induced by repeated cycles of low-calorie dieting in which the body prepares itself for famine. Because meals are coming at shorter, regular intervals, your body learns to process food more efficiently, and your metabolism is accelerated as a result.

Avoid Fat-Producing Foods.

As mentioned, certain foods can be easily converted to fat in the body, making them a poor choice for bodybuilders. Diets high in simple sugars, for example, stimulate certain fat-producing enzymes in the body and cause an overproduction of insulin, which leads to excess fat storage. Any food that promotes body fat also impedes muscular growth.

Fruits and fruit juices should also be avoided if you're trying to stay lean. Though healthy and high in vitamins, minerals, and fiber, fruits and fruit juices are composed largely of the simple sugar fructose. Because of its unique molecular structure, fructose is converted to a long-chain triglyceride (fat) in the liver. Much of the innocent fruit you eat ends up in the bloodstream as fat. By eliminating fruit

Dietary control of metabolism is important to great pros like J. J. Marsh. Photo by J. M. Manion.

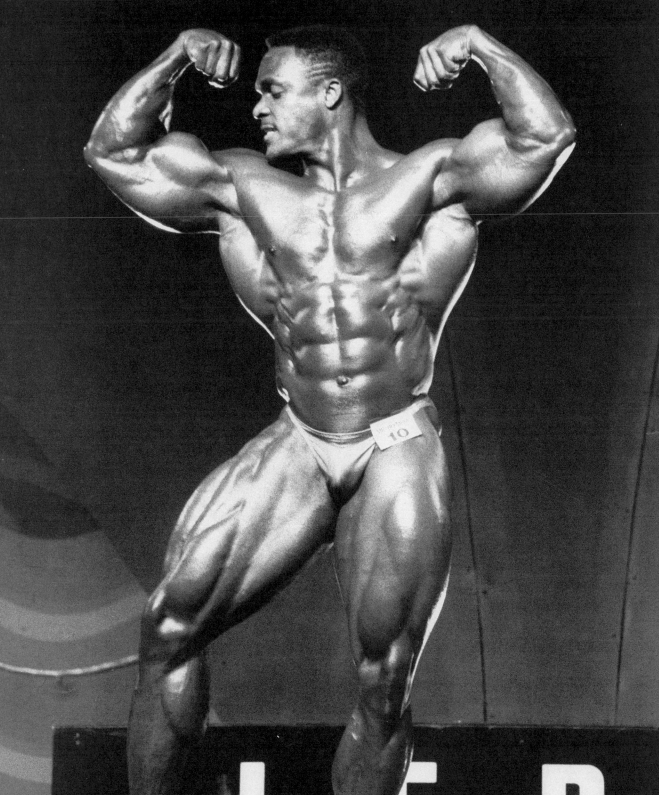

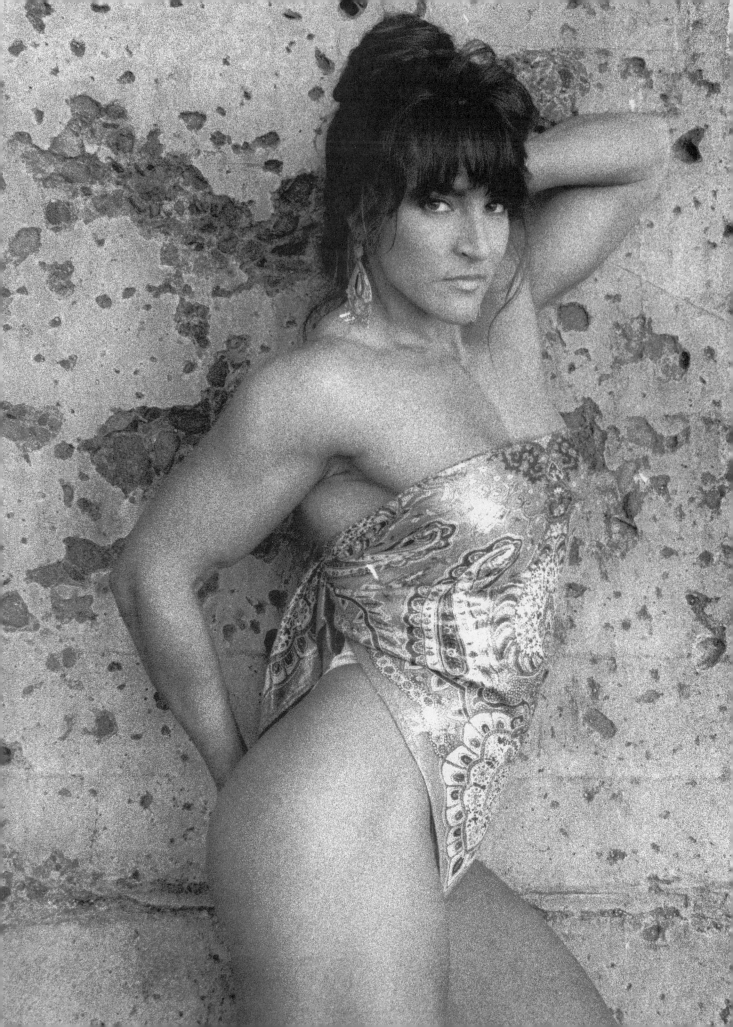

from your diet, you can get leaner and much more defined.

Dairy products are another food to avoid.* In addition to being high in fat, dairy products contain the milk sugar lactose, another simple sugar that can be readily converted to body fat. Not only that, dairy products can cause allergic reactions such as water retention and puffiness in susceptible individuals. Even though dairy products supply the bone-building mineral calcium, you can obtain an ample supply of calcium from vegetables and nutritional supplements. A cup of kale, for example, has nearly as much calcium as an eight-ounce glass of milk.

Practice Nutritional Supplementation.

When people first hear that my nutrition program allows up to 10,000 calories a day or more, they are amazed. But not all of those calories come from food. A certain proportion comes from nutritional supplements. If you're eating 10,000 calories a day, for example, about 4,000 of those calories are usually obtained from food supplements such as medium-chain fatty acids (MCFAs) and protein and carbohydrate supplements.

Nutritional supplements play a key role in metabolism and nutrition. Used in conjunction with the proper foods, they assist in decreasing body fat, supporting muscular growth, extending endurance, and promoting better recovery and repair after training.

At this point, I hope you understand the fundamental metabolic principles behind my nutrition program. Now, let's take a look at how you can tailor this information to plan meals for optimum results.

*Growing children and teenagers and pregnant and lactating women should not restrict dairy products.

Lisa Lorio knows that proper nutrition is the foundation of bodybuilding success. Photo by Paul B. Goode.

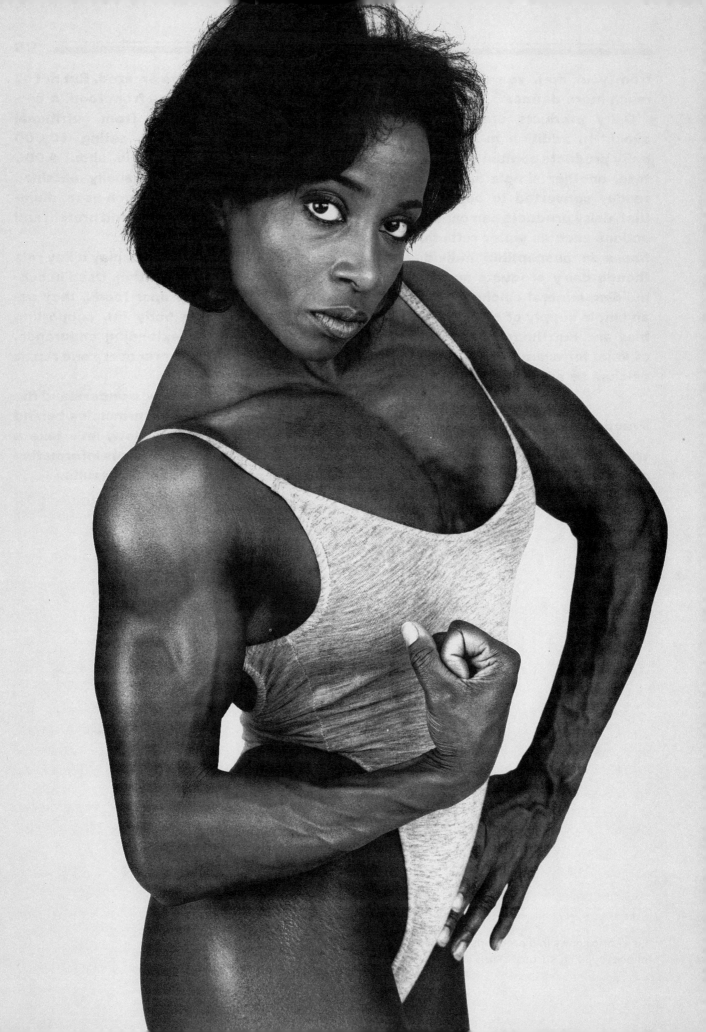

THREE
PLANNING FOR PERFECTION

Where can you make the most dramatic changes in the way you look? If you're like most people, you probably answered "in the gym." Not true! The most dramatic changes you make in your physique start in the kitchen—with the foods you prepare and eat. Nutrition is the single most important variable in bodybuilding. All the weight training and aerobic exercise in the world won't do a bit of good unless you're fueling yourself properly with the right foods and nutritional supplements, in the right amounts and combinations.

While following this nutrition program, you should keep accurate records of everything you eat, including the supplements you take. To do this, you'll need a nutrition diary (see Appendix C), a food scale to weigh your portions, and a food composition guide that provides information on the nutrient values of foods. On your nutrition diary, record the date, your body weight, time, foods, and the nutritional values of those foods. If you wish, use the back of the sheet to make notes about how you look and feel each day.

Bodybuilding great Carla Dunlap is one of the sport's most enduring athletes. Photo by Paul B. Goode.

BASIC MEAL PLANNING

On my nutrition program, women eat between 2,000 and 6,000 calories a day; and men, between 6,000 and 10,000 calories a day or more. To begin the program, you need a caloric base from which you can build, adding more calories. This base varies from person to person and depends on how many calories you now average and somewhat on what you weigh. Some women, for example, may be eating only 1,500 or 1,800 calories a day, and so beginning the program at 3,000 calories would be foolish. A starting point of 2,000 calories would be more sensible. In other words, you should not jump in at the upper caloric levels because you could have a difficult time consuming such a large quantity of food.

Here are step-by-step guidelines on how to plan your daily menus:

1. Decide on how many calories you require per meal. Select your caloric base, and divide that number by the number of daily meals you'll eat, five, six, or more. This gives you the approximate number of calories to eat at each meal.

For example, if your caloric base is

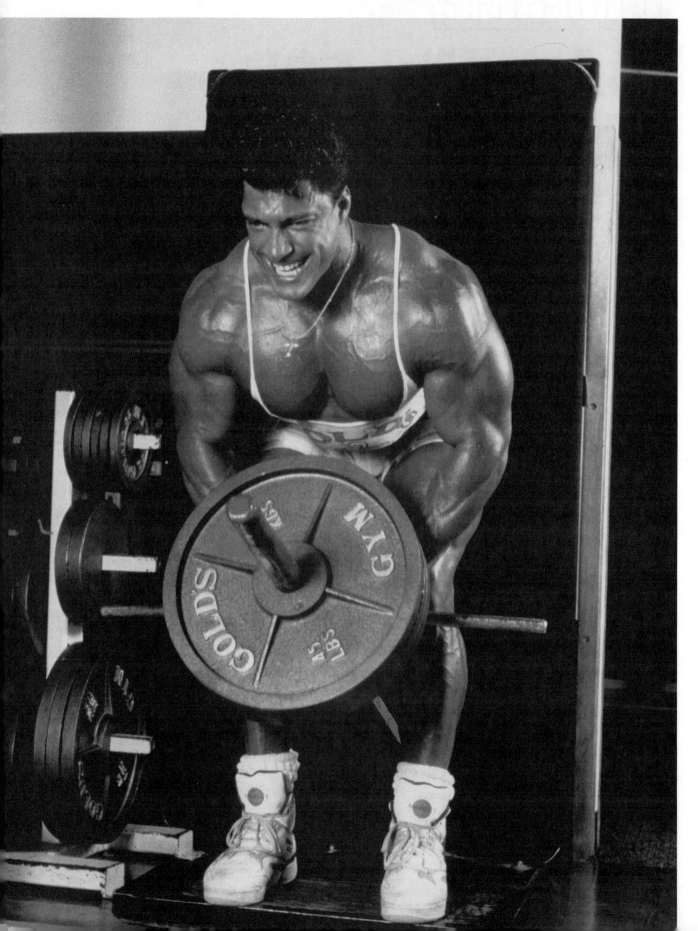

Bob Cicherillo is a hot phenomenon in bodybuilding.
Photo by Jim Amentler.

5,000 calories and you plan to eat six meals a day, each meal should provide approximately 833 calories.

2. Choose protein sources. Next, determine how much protein you need to meet your daily protein requirements. Each day you should eat 1.25 to 1.5 grams of protein per pound of body weight. At least one gram of protein per pound of your body weight should come from complete protein sources such as lean white-meat poultry, fish, egg whites, or protein powder. The remaining should come from starchy and fibrous carbohydrates, which also contain protein. To determine the exact amount of protein to consume, use the following equation:

Your body weight × 1.5 (or 1.25) = Required grams of protein per day. (Someone who weighs 175 pounds, for example, would need 262.5 grams of protein a day.)

Divide your daily protein intake by the number of daily meals to calculate how many grams of protein you need at each of those meals.

4. Choose Carbohydrates. Decide which fibrous carbohydrates you'll eat and how many grams of each. Figure in one or two per meal. At this point, subtotal your calories to see how much you have left to "spend" on starchy carbohydrates. Figure in one or two starchy carbohydrates a meal.

5. Add in calories from supplements. To increase your daily caloric intake, use supplements. The supplements I recommend are a carbohydrate supplement, a protein powder or protein/carbohydrate bar, and a medium-chain fatty acids (MCFAs) supplement, also known as MCT oil. More information on protein and carbohydrate supplements is available in Chapter 4, and guidelines for using MCFAs are provided in Chapter 5.

MEAL PREPARATION

Once you know what foods to eat and how many grams of each, you are ready to prepare your meals. Using a food scale, weigh the food in its raw or frozen form, not after it has been cooked. That way, you'll be more accurate because cooking can reduce the weight of food without changing its caloric content.

Lean proteins should be baked, broiled, microwaved, or grilled—without fats; and vegetables should be microwaved, lightly steamed, or cooked in a minimal amount of water to preserve nutrient content. Whenever possible, eat fibrous carbohydrates raw because they are more nutritious that way. In Appendix B, you'll find some delicious recipes you can incorporate in your meal planning.

Eating the same foods day after day leads to boredom, and in some people, allergies. By eating a variety of foods daily, you will get a better balance of nutrients. That's why it's a good idea to bulk-prepare a variety of foods, store them in containers, and refrigerate or freeze them until ready to eat.

SAMPLE MENUS

To help you plan your own menus, here are some samples you can follow:*

*Nutrient values of the menus in this book have been calculated using Parrillo Performance products, including Hi-Protein Powder™, Pro-Carb™, The Bar™, and CapTri®, a medium-chain fatty-acid oil. Other products may yield different calculations.

2,000 CALORIES

Sample Weight: 115

Time/Food	Amt.	Calories	Protein/g	Fat/g	Carbs/g	Na/mg	K/mg
8 A.M.							
Protein Pwd.	1 Scp.	105	20.0	1.0	6.0	125	50
Oatmeal	50 g.	195	7.1	3.7	34.1	1	176
Egg whites	100 g.	51	10.9	0.0	0.8	146	139
MCFA Oil	0.5 Tbsp.	57					
Subtotal		408	38.0	4.7	40.9	272	365
11 A.M.							
Chicken	75 g.	88	17.6	1.4	0.0	38	240
Potato	25 g.	19	0.5	0.0	17.1	1	88
Asparagus	25 g.	7	0.6	0.1	1.3	1	70
Salad	300 g.	69	3.3	0.3	14.4	48	780
MCFA Oil	1 Tbsp.	114					
Subtotal		296	22.0	1.8	32.7	87	1,178
1 P.M.							
Halibut	100 g.	100	20.9	1.2	0.0	54	449
Brown Rice	25 g.	90	1.9	0.5	19.4	2	54
Corn	25 g.	24	0.9	0.3	5.5	0	70
Green Beans	25 g.	8	0.5	0.1	1.8	2	61
MCFA Oil	0.5 Tbsp.	57					
Subtotal		279	24.1	2.0	26.7	58	633
3 P.M.							
Haddock	125 g.	99	22.9	0.1	0.0	76	380
Black-eyed Peas	25 g.	33	2.3	0.1	5.9	13	97
Broccoli	25 g.	8	0.9	0.1	1.5	4	71
Salad	300 g.	69	3.3	0.3	14.4	48	780
MCFA Oil	1 Tbsp.	114					
Subtotal		323	29.3	0.6	21.8	141	1,327
Carbohydrate Supplement (during and after workout)							
	2 Scps.	210	8.0	0.0	44.0	128	344
6 P.M.							
Cod	125 g.	98	22.0	0.4	0.0	89	478
Sweet Potato	25 g.	29	0.4	0.1	6.6	3	61
Cauliflower	25 g.	7	0.7	0.1	1.3	3	74
Lima Beans	25 g.	26	1.6	0.0	4.9	32	123
Salad	300 g.	69	3.3	0.3	14.4	48	780
MCFA Oil	0.5 Tbsp.	57					
Subtotal		284	28.0	0.9	27.2	175	1,515
8 P.M.							
Turkey Breast	75 g.	87	18.5	0.9	0.0	38	240
Potato	50 g.	38	1.1	0.1	34.1	1	176
Zucchini	25 g.	4	0.3	0.0	0.9	0	51
Salad	300 g	69	3.3	0.3	14.4	48	780
MCFA Oil	0.5 Tbsp.	57					
Subtotal		255	23.1	1.3	49.4	88	1,247
Daily Totals		2,055	172.5	11.2	242.6	947	6,608

Athena is a bodybuilder and fitness model from New York City. Photo by Jimmie D. King.

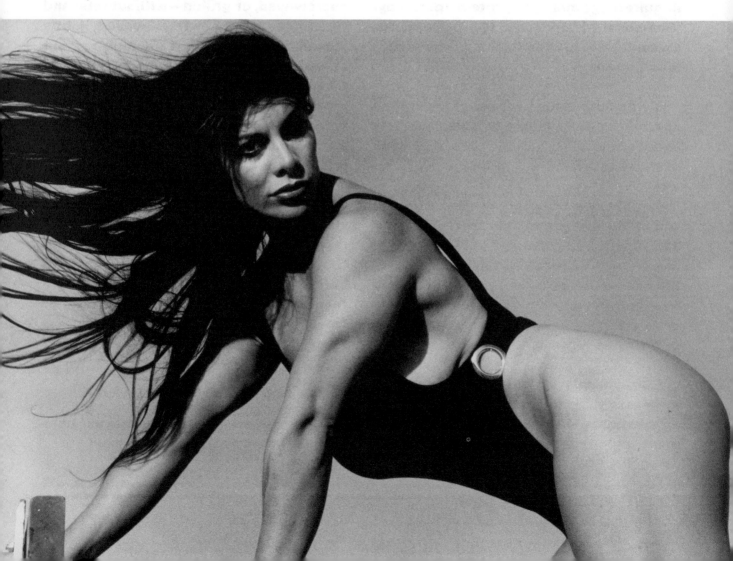

3,000 CALORIES

Sample Weight: 145

Time/Food	Amt.	Calories	Protein/g	Fat/g	Carbs/g	Na/mg	K/mg
8 A.M.							
Protein Pwd.	1 Scp.	105	20.0	1.0	6.0	125	50
Oatmeal	50 g.	195	7.1	3.7	34.1	1	176
Egg whites	100 g.	51	10.9	0.0	0.8	146	139
MCFA Oil	1 Tbsp.	114					
Subtotal		465	38.0	4.7	40.9	272	365
11 A.M.							
Chicken Breast	125 g.	146	29.3	2.4	0.0	63	400
Potato	100 g.	76	2.1	0.1	68.2	2	352
Asparagus	50 g.	13	1.3	0.1	2.5	1	139
Salad	300 g.	69	3.3	0.3	14.4	48	780
MCFA Oil	1 Tbsp.	114					
Subtotal		418	35.9	2.9	85.1	114	1,671
1 P.M.							
Halibut	125 g.	125	26.1	1.5	0.0	68	561
Brown Rice	50 g.	180	3.8	1.0	38.8	5	107
Corn	50 g.	48	1.8	0.5	11.1	0	140
Green Beans	75 g.	24	1.4	0.2	5.3	5	182
MCFA Oil	1 Tbsp.	114					
Subtotal		491	33.1	3.1	55.2	77	991
3 P.M.							
Haddock	125 g.	99	22.9	0.1	0.0	76	380
Black-eyed Peas	100 g.	131	9.0	0.4	23.6	50	387
Broccoli	50 g.	16	1.8	0.2	3.0	8	141
Salad	300 g.	69	3.3	0.3	14.4	48	780
MCFA Oil	1 Tbsp.	114					
Subtotal		429	37.0	1.0	41.0	182	1,688
Protein/Carbohydrate Bar (after workout)							
	1 Bar	240	11.0	1.0	38.0	50	210
6 P.M.							
Cod	125 g.	98	22.0	0.4	0.0	89	478
Sweet Potato	100 g.	114	1.7	0.4	26.3	10	243
Cauliflower	25 g.	7	0.7	0.1	1.3	3	74
Lima Beans	50 g.	51	3.1	0.1	9.8	65	245
Salad	300 g.	69	3.3	0.3	14.4	48	780
MCFA Oil	1 Tbsp.	114					
Subtotal		452	30.8	1.2	51.8	215	1,819
8 P.M.							
Turkey Breast	100 g.	116	24.6	1.2	0.0	51	320
Potato	125 g.	95	2.6	0.1	85.3	3	440
Zucchini	50 g.	9	0.6	0.1	1.8	1	101
Salad	300 g.	69	3.3	0.3	14.4	48	780
MCFA Oil	1.5 Tbsp.	171					
Subtotal		460	31.1	1.7	101.5	102	1,641
Daily Totals		2,955	216.8	15.5	413.3	1,011	8,385

4,000 CALORIES

Sample Weight: 160

Time/Food	Amt.	Calories	Protein/g	Fat/g	Carbs/g	Na/mg	K/mg
8 A.M.							
Protein Pwd.	1 Scp.	105	20.0	1.0	6.0	125	50
Oatmeal	100 g.	390	14.2	7.4	68.2	2	352
Egg whites	100 g.	51	10.9	0.0	0.8	146	139
MCFA Oil	2 Tbsp.	228					
Subtotal		774	45.1	8.4	75.0	273	541
11 A.M.							
Chicken Breast	150 g.	176	35.1	2.9	0.0	75	480
Potato	125 g.	95	2.6	0.1	85.3	3	440
Asparagus	50 g.	13	1.3	0.1	2.5	1	139
Salad	300 g.	69	3.3	0.3	14.4	48	780
MCFA Oil	2 Tbsp.	228					
Subtotal		581	42.3	3.4	102.2	127	1,839

Time/Food	Amt.	Calories	Protein/g	Fat/g	Carbs/g	Na/mg	K/mg
1 P.M.							
Halibut	125 g.	125	26.1	1.5	0.0	68	561
Brown Rice	100 g.	360	7.5	1.9	77.6	9	214
Corn	50 g.	48	1.8	0.5	11.1	0	140
Green Beans	75 g.	24	1.4	0.2	5.3	5	182
MCFA Oil	1 Tbsp.	114					
Subtotal		671	36.8	4.1	94.0	82	1,098
3 P.M.							
Haddock	125 g.	99	22.9	0.1	0.0	76	380
Black-eyed Peas	100 g.	131	9.0	0.4	23.6	50	387
Broccoli	75 g.	24	2.7	0.2	4.4	11	212
Salad	300 g.	69	3.3	0.3	14.4	48	780
MCFA Oil	2 Tbsp.	228					
Subtotal		551	37.9	1.1	42.4	186	1,759
Protein/Carbohydrate Bar (after workout)							
	1 Bar	240	11.0	1.0	38.0	50	210
6 P.M.							
Cod	125 g.	98	22.0	0.4	0.0	89	478
Sweet Potato	100 g.	114	1.7	0.4	26.3	10	243
Cauliflower	50 g.	14	1.4	0.1	2.6	7	148
Lima Beans	75 g.	77	4.7	0.1	14.6	97	368
Salad	300 g.	69	3.3	0.3	14.4	48	780
MCFA Oil	2 Tbsp.	228					
Subtotal		599	33.0	1.3	57.9	250	2,016
8 P.M.							
Turkey Breast	100 g.	116	24.6	1.2	0.0	51	320
Potato	175 g.	133	3.7	0.2	119.4	4	616
Zucchini	100 g.	17	1.2	0.1	3.6	1	202
Salad	300 g.	69	3.3	0.3	14.4	48	780
MCFA Oil	2 Tbsp.	228					
Subtotal		563	32.8	1.8	137.4	104	1,918
Daily Totals		3,978	238.8	20.9	546.8	1070	9,380

5,000 CALORIES

Sample Weight: 172

Time/Food	Amt.	Calories	Protein/g	Fat/g	Carbs/g	Na/mg	K/mg
8 A.M.							
Protein Pwd.	1 Scp.	105	20.0	1.0	6.0	125	50
Corn Grits	100 g.	362	8.7	0.8	78.1	1	80
Egg whites	100 g.	51	10.9	0.0	0.8	146	139
MCFA Oil	2 Tbsp.	228					
Subtotal		746	39.6	1.8	84.9	272	269
11 A.M.							
Chicken Breast	150 g.	176	35.1	2.9	0.0	75	480
Potato	175 g.	133	3.7	0.2	119.4	4	616
Asparagus	100 g.	26	2.5	0.2	5.0	2	278
Salad	300 g.	69	3.3	0.3	14.4	48	780
MCFA Oil	3 Tbsp.	342					
Subtotal		746	44.6	3.5	138.8	129	2,154
1 P.M.							
Halibut	125 g.	125	26.1	1.5	0.0	68	561
Brown Rice	100 g.	360	7.5	1.9	77.6	9	214
Corn	75 g.	72	2.6	0.8	16.6	0	210
Green Beans	125 g.	40	2.4	0.3	8.9	9	304
MCFA Oil	2 Tbsp.	228					
Subtotal		825	38.6	4.4	103.1	85	1,289
3 P.M.							
Haddock	150 g.	119	27.5	0.2	0.0	92	456
Black-eyed Peas	150 g.	197	13.5	0.6	35.4	75	581
Broccoli	100 g.	32	3.6	0.3	5.9	15	282
Salad	300 g.	69	3.3	0.3	14.4	48	780
MCFA Oil	3 Tbsp.	342					
Subtotal		758	47.9	1.4	55.7	230	2,099
Protein/Carbohydrate Bar (after workout)							
	2 Bars	480	22.0	2.0	76.0	100	420

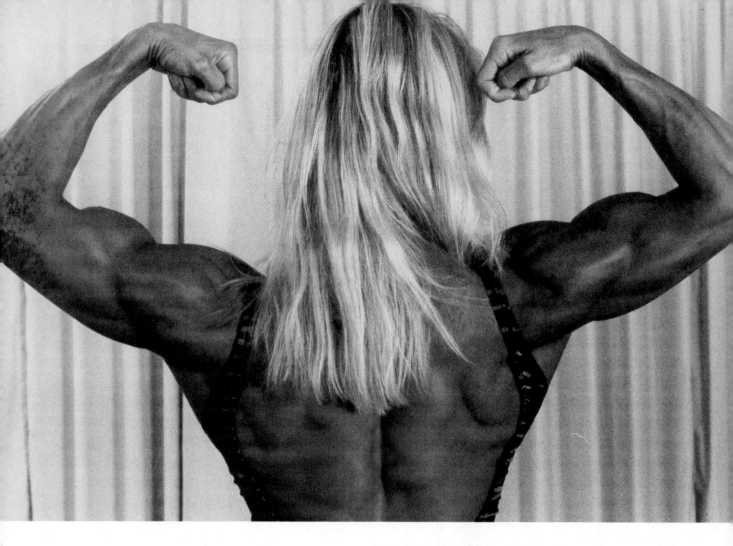

Kathy Unger's back is ripped to the max. Photo by Jimmie D. King.

5,000 CALORIES *(Continued)*

Time/Food	Amt.	Calories	Protein/g	Fat/g	Carbs/g	Na/mg	K/mg
6 P.M.							
Cod	125 g.	98	22.0	0.4	0.0	89	478
Sweet Potato	150 g.	171	2.6	0.6	39.5	15	365
Cauliflower	100 g.	27	2.7	0.2	5.2	13	295
Lima Beans	75 g.	77	4.7	0.1	14.6	97	368
Salad	300 g.	69	3.3	0.3	14.4	48	780
MCFA Oil	3 Tbsp.	342					
Subtotal		783	35.2	1.6	73.7	262	2,285
8 P.M.							
Turkey Breast	100 g.	116	24.6	1.2	0.0	51	320
Potato	200 g.	152	4.2	0.2	136.4	4	704
Zucchini	125 g.	21	1.5	0.1	4.5	1	253
Salad	300 g.	69	3.3	0.3	14.4	48	780
MCFA Oil	3 Tbsp.	342					
Subtotal		700	33.6	1.8	155.3	104	2,057
Daily Totals		5,038	261.5	16.5	687.4	1181	10,572

6,000 CALORIES

Sample Weight: 185

Time/Food	Amt.	Calories	Protein/g	Fat/g	Carbs/g	Na/mg	K/mg
8 A.M.							
Protein Pwd.	1 Scp.	105	20.0	1.0	6.0	125	50
Shredded Wheat	100 g.	354	9.9	2.0	79.9	3	348
Egg whites	100 g.	51	10.9	0.0	0.8	146	139
MCFA Oil	4 Tbsp.	456					
Subtotal		966	40.8	3.0	86.7	274	537

Time/Food	Amt.	Calories	Protein/g	Fat/g	Carbs/g	Na/mg	K/mg
11 A.M.							
Chicken Breast	150 g.	176	35.1	2.9	0.0	75	480
Potato	225 g.	171	4.7	0.2	153.5	5	792
Asparagus	125 g.	33	3.1	0.3	6.3	3	348
Salad	300 g.	69	3.3	0.3	14.4	48	780
MCFA Oil	3.5 Tbsp	399					
Subtotal		847	46.3	3.6	174.1	130	2,400
1 P.M.							
Halibut	125 g.	125	26.1	1.5	0.0	68	561
Brown Rice	150 g.	540	11.3	2.9	116.4	14	321
Corn	150 g.	144	5.3	1.5	33.2	0	420
Green Beans	75 g.	24	1.4	0.2	5.3	5	182
MCFA Oil	3 Tbsp.	342					
Subtotal		1,175	44.1	6.0	154.9	86	1,485
3 P.M.							
Haddock	150 g.	119	27.5	0.2	0.0	92	456
Black-eyed Peas	200 g.	262	18.0	0.8	47.2	100	774
Broccoli	150 g.	48	5.4	0.5	8.9	23	423
Salad	300 g.	69	3.3	0.3	14.4	48	780
MCFA Oil	3 Tbsp.	342					
Subtotal		840	54.2	1.7	70.5	262	2,433
Protein/Carbohydrate Bar (after workout)							
	2 Bars	480	22.0	2.0	76.0	100	420

6,000 CALORIES *(Continued)*

Time/Food	Amt.	Calories	Protein/g	Fat/g	Carbs/g	Na/mg	K/mg
6 P.M.							
Cod	125 g.	98	22.0	0.4	0.0	89	478
Sweet Potato	200 g.	228	3.4	0.8	52.6	20	486
Cauliflower	125 g.	34	3.4	0.3	6.5	16	369
Lima Beans	150 g.	153	9.3	0.2	29.3	194	735
Salad	300 g.	69	3.3	0.3	14.4	48	780
MCFA Oil	3 Tbsp.	342					
Subtotal		923	41.4	1.9	102.8	367	2,847
8 P.M.							
Turkey Breast	100 g.	116	24.6	1.2	0.0	51	320
Potato	200 g.	152	4.2	0.2	136.4	4	704
Zucchini	175 g.	30	2.1	0.2	6.3	2	354
Salad	300 g.	69	3.3	0.3	14.4	48	780
MCFA Oil	3.5 Tbsp.	399					
Subtotal		766	34.2	1.9	157.1	105	2,158
Daily Totals		5,997	282.8	20.1	822.0	1,324	12,279

7,000 CALORIES

Sample Weight: 200

Time/Food	Amt.	Calories	Protein/g	Fat/g	Carbs/g	Na/mg	K/mg
8 A.M.							
Protein Pwd.	1 Scp.	105	20.0	1.0	6.0	125	50
Oatmeal	125 g.	488	17.8	9.3	85.3	3	440
Egg whites	100 g.	51	10.9	0.0	0.8	146	139
MCFA Oil	4 Tbsp.	456					
Subtotal		1,100	48.7	10.3	92.1	274	629
11 A.M.							
Chicken Breast	150 g.	176	35.1	2.9	0.0	75	480
Potato	275 g.	209	5.8	0.3	187.6	6	968
Asparagus	200 g.	52	5.0	0.4	10.0	4	556
Salad	400 g.	92	4.4	0.4	19.2	64	1,040
MCFA Oil	4 Tbsp.	456					
Subtotal		985	50.3	3.9	216.8	149	3,044
1 P.M.							
Halibut	125 g.	125	26.1	1.5	0.0	68	561
Brown Rice	175 g.	630	13.1	3.3	135.8	16	375
Corn	175 g.	168	6.1	1.8	38.7	0	490
Green Beans	125 g.	40	2.4	0.3	8.9	9	304
MCFA Oil	4 Tbsp.	456					
Subtotal		1,419	47.8	6.8	183.4	92	1,730
3 P.M.							
Haddock	125 g.	99	22.9	0.1	0.0	76	380
Black-eyed Peas	225 g.	295	20.3	0.9	53.1	113	871
Broccoli	225 g.	72	8.1	0.7	13.3	34	635
Salad	400 g.	92	4.4	0.4	19.2	64	1,040
MCFA Oil	4 Tbsp.	456					
Subtotal		1,014	55.6	2.1	85.6	287	2,925
Protein/Carbohydrate Bar (after workout)							
	2 Bars	480	22.0	2.0	76.0	100	420
6 P.M.							
Cod	125 g.	98	22.0	0.4	0.0	89	478
Sweet Potato	250 g.	285	4.3	1.0	65.8	25	608
Cauliflower	175 g.	47	4.7	0.4	9.1	23	516
Lima Beans	175 g.	179	10.9	0.2	34.1	226	858
Salad	400 g.	92	4.4	0.4	19.2	64	1,040
MCFA Oil	4 Tbsp.	456					
Subtotal		1,156	46.2	2.3	128.2	426	3,499
8 P.M.							
Turkey Breast	125 g.	145	30.8	1.5	0.0	64	400
Potato	250 g.	190	5.3	0.3	170.5	5	880
Zucchini	200 g.	34	2.4	0.2	7.2	2	404
Peas	75 g.	55	4.1	0.2	9.6	97	113
MCFA Oil	4 Tbsp.	456					
Subtotal		880	42.5	2.2	187.3	168	1,797
Daily Totals		7,033	313.0	29.6	969.2	1,494	14,043

8,000 CALORIES

Sample Weight: 210

Time/Food	Amt.	Calories	Protein/g	Fat/g	Carbs/g	Na/mg	K/mg
8 A.M.							
Protein Pwd.	1 Scp.	105	20.0	1.0	6.0	125	50
Oatmeal	125 g.	488	17.8	9.3	85.3	3	440
Egg whites	100 g.	51	10.9	0.0	0.8	146	139
MCFA Oil	5 Tbsp.	570					
Subtotal		1,214	48.7	10.3	92.1	274	629
11 A.M.							
Chicken Breast	150 g.	176	35.1	2.9	0.0	75	480
Potato	300 g.	228	6.3	0.3	204.6	6	1,056
Asparagus	200 g.	52	5.0	0.4	10.0	4	556
Salad	400 g.	92	4.4	0.4	19.2	64	1,040
MCFA Oil	5 Tbsp.	570					
Subtotal		1,118	50.8	4.0	233.8	149	3,132
1 P.M.							
Halibut	125 g.	125	26.1	1.5	0.0	68	561
Brown Rice	200 g.	720	15.0	3.8	155.2	18	428
Corn	200 g.	192	7.0	2.0	44.2	0	560
Green Beans	125 g.	40	2.4	0.3	8.9	9	304
MCFA Oil	4.5 Tbsp.	513					
Subtotal		1,590	50.5	7.6	208.3	94	1,853
3 P.M.							
Haddock	25 g.	99	22.9	0.1	0.0	76	380
Black-eyed Peas	275 g.	360	24.8	1.1	64.9	138	1,064
Broccoli	225 g.	72	8.1	0.7	13.3	34	635
Salad	400 g.	92	4.4	0.4	19.2	64	1,040
MCFA Oil	5 Tbsp.	570					
Subtotal		1,193	60.1	2.3	97.4	312	3,119
Protein/Carbohydrate Bar (after workout)							
	2 Bars	480	22.0	2.0	76.0	100	420
6 P.M.							
Cod	125 g.	98	22.0	0.4	0.0	89	478
Sweet Potato	300 g.	342	5.1	1.2	78.9	30	729
Cauliflower	175 g.	47	4.7	0.4	9.1	23	516
Lima Beans	225 g.	230	14.0	0.2	43.9	290	1,103
Salad	400 g.	92	4.4	0.4	19.2	64	1,040
MCFA Oil	4.5 Tbsp.	513					
Subtotal		1,321	50.2	2.6	151.1	496	3,865
8 P.M.							
Turkey Breast	125 g.	145	30.8	1.5	0.0	64	400
Potato	325 g.	247	6.8	0.3	221.7	7	1,144
Zucchini	200 g.	34	2.4	0.2	7.2	2	404
Peas	125 g.	91	6.8	0.4	16.0	161	188
MCFA Oil	5 Tbsp.	570					
Subtotal		1,087	46.7	2.4	244.9	234	2,136
Daily Totals		8,003	329.0	31.0	1,103.4	1,658	15,154

9,000 CALORIES

Sample Weight: 220

Time/Food	Amt.	Calories	Protein/g	Fat/g	Carbs/g	Na/mg	K/mg
8 A.M.							
Protein Pwd.	1 Scp.	105	20.0	1.0	6.0	125	50
Oatmeal	175 g.	683	24.9	13.0	119.4	4	616
Egg whites	100 g.	51	10.9	0.0	0.8	146	139
MCFA Oil	5 Tbsp	570					
Subtotal		1,409	55.8	14.0	126.2	275	805
11 A.M.							
Chicken Breast	150 g.	176	35.1	2.9	0.0	75	480
Potato	375 g.	285	7.9	0.4	255.8	8	1,320
Asparagus	225 g.	59	5.6	0.5	11.3	5	626
Salad	400 g.	92	4.4	0.4	19.2	64	1,040
MCFA Oil	6 Tbsp	684					
Subtotal		1,295	53.0	4.1	286.2	151	3,466

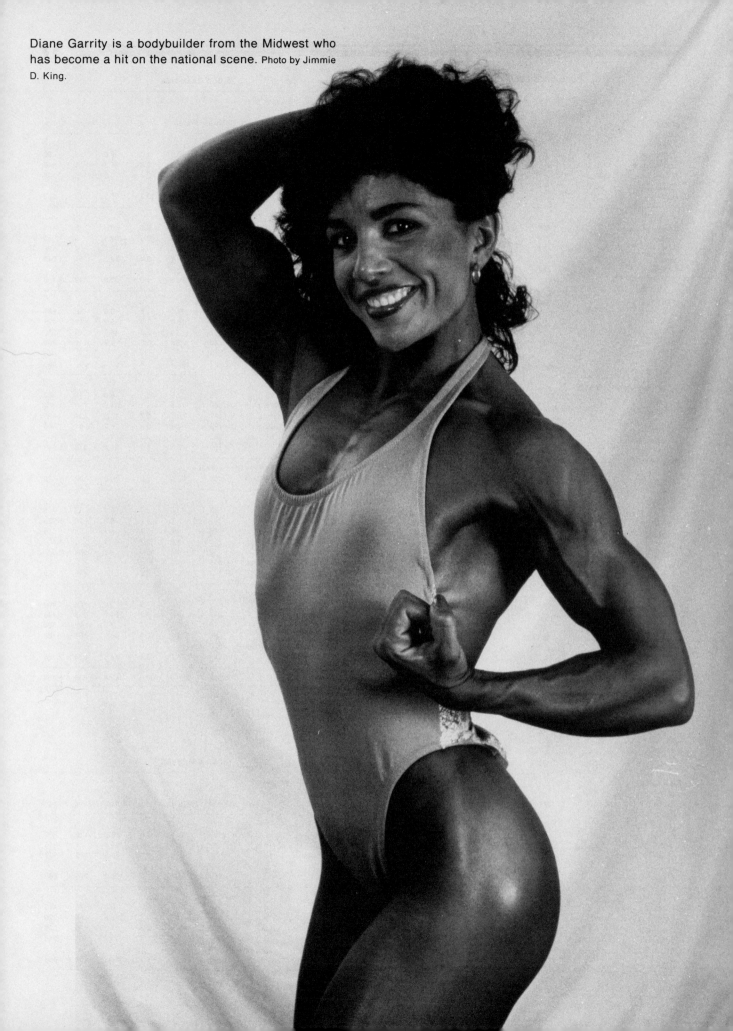

Diane Garrity is a bodybuilder from the Midwest who has become a hit on the national scene. Photo by Jimmie D. King.

9,000 CALORIES (Continued)

Time/Food	Amt.	Calories	Protein/g	Fat/g	Carbs/g	Na/mg	K/mg
1 P.M.							
Halibut	125 g.	125	26.1	1.5	0.0	68	561
Brown Rice	225 g.	810	16.9	4.3	174.6	20	482
Corn	200 g.	192	7.0	2.0	44.2	0	560
Green Beans	125 g.	40	2.4	0.3	8.9	9	304
MCFA Oil	5 Tbsp.	570					
Subtotal		1,737	52.4	8.0	227.7	97	1,907
3 P.M.							
Haddock	125 g.	99	22.9	0.1	0.0	76	380
Black-eyed Peas	325 g.	426	29.3	1.3	76.7	163	1,258
Broccoli	225 g.	72	8.1	0.7	13.3	34	635
Salad	400 g.	92	4.4	0.4	19.2	64	1,040
MCFA Oil	6 Tbsp.	684					
Subtotal		1,373	64.6	2.5	109.2	337	3,312
Protein/Carbohydrate Bar (after workout)							
	2 Bars	480	22.0	2.0	76.0	100	420
6 P.M.							
Cod	125 g.	98	22.0	0.4	0.0	89	478
Sweet Potato	350 g.	399	6.0	1.4	92.1	35	851
Cauliflower	175 g.	47	4.7	0.4	9.1	23	516
Lima Beans	225 g.	230	14.0	0.2	43.9	290	1,103
Salad	400 g.	92	4.4	0.4	19.2	64	1,040
MCFA Oil	5 Tbsp.	570					
Subtotal		1,435	51.0	2.8	164.2	501	3,987
8 P.M.							
Turkey Breast	125 g.	145	30.8	1.5	0.0	64	400
Potato	400 g.	304	8.4	0.4	272.8	8	1,408
Zucchini	200 g.	34	2.4	0.2	7.2	2	404
Peas	150 g.	110	8.1	0.5	19.2	194	225
MCFA Oil	6 Tbsp.	684					
Subtotal		1,277	49.7	2.6	299.2	267	2,437
Daily Totals		9,005	348.4	35.9	1,288.6	1,727	16,333

Time/Food	Amt.	Calories	Protein/g	Fat/g	Carbs/g	Na/mg	K/mg
6 P.M.							
Cod	125 g.	98	22.0	0.4	0.0	89	478
Sweet Potato	450 g.	513	7.7	1.8	118.4	45	1,094
Cauliflower	175 g.	47	4.7	0.4	9.1	23	516
Lima Beans	225 g.	230	14.0	0.2	43.9	290	1,103
Salad	400 g.	92	4.4	0.4	19.2	64	1,040
MCFA Oil	5.5 Tbsp.	627					
Subtotal		1,606	52.7	3.2	190.5	511	4,230
8 P.M.							
Turkey Breast	125 g.	145	30.8	1.5	0.0	64	400
Potato	475 g.	361	10.0	0.5	324.0	10	1,672
Zucchini	200 g.	34	2.4	0.2	7.2	2	404
Peas	175 g.	128	9.5	0.5	22.4	226	263
MCFA Oil	6 Tbsp.	684					
Subtotal		1,352	52.6	2.7	353.6	301	2,739
Daily Totals		9,965	360.2	38.4	1,478.3	1,954	17,779

THE NEXT STEP

I've already mentioned the importance of using supplements as an adjunct to proper nutrition. Now it's time to cover the specifics of supplementation. In the next two chapters, I explain exactly which supplements work most effectively and how to use them in my nutrition program.

10,000 CALORIES

Sample Weight: 230

Time/Food	Amt.	Calories	Protein/g	Fat/g	Carbs/g	Na/mg	K/mg
8 A.M.							
Protein Pwd.	1 Scp.	105	20.0	1.0	6.0	125	50
Oatmeal	225 g.	878	32.0	16.7	153.5	5	792
Egg whites	100 g.	51	10.9	0.0	0.8	146	139
MCFA Oil	6 Tbsp.	684					
Subtotal		1,718	62.9	17.7	160.3	276	981
11 A.M.							
Chicken Breast	150 g.	176	35.1	2.9	0.0	75	480
Potato	450 g.	342	9.5	0.5	306.9	9	1,584
Asparagus	225 g.	59	5.6	0.5	11.3	5	626
Salad	400 g.	92	4.4	0.4	19.2	64	1,040
MCFA Oil	7 Tbsp.	798					
Subtotal		1,466	54.6	4.2	337.4	153	3,730
1 P.M.							
Halibut	125 g.	125	26.1	1.5	0.0	68	561
Brown Rice	225 g.	810	16.9	4.3	174.6	20	482
Corn	200 g.	192	7.0	2.0	44.2	0	560
Green Beans	125 g.	40	2.4	0.3	8.9	9	304
MCFA Oil	6 Tbsp.	684					
Subtotal		1,851	52.4	8.0	227.7	97	1,907
3 P.M.							
Haddock	125 g.	99	22.9	0.1	0.0	76	380
Black-eyed Peas	375 g.	491	33.8	1.5	88.5	188	1,451
Broccoli	225 g.	72	8.1	0.7	13.3	34	635
Salad	400 g.	92	4.4	0.4	19.2	64	1,040
MCFA Oil	7 Tbsp.	798					
Subtotal		1,552	69.1	2.7	121.0	362	3,506
Carbohydrate Supplement (during and after workout)							
	4 Scps.	420	16.0	0.0	88.0	256	688

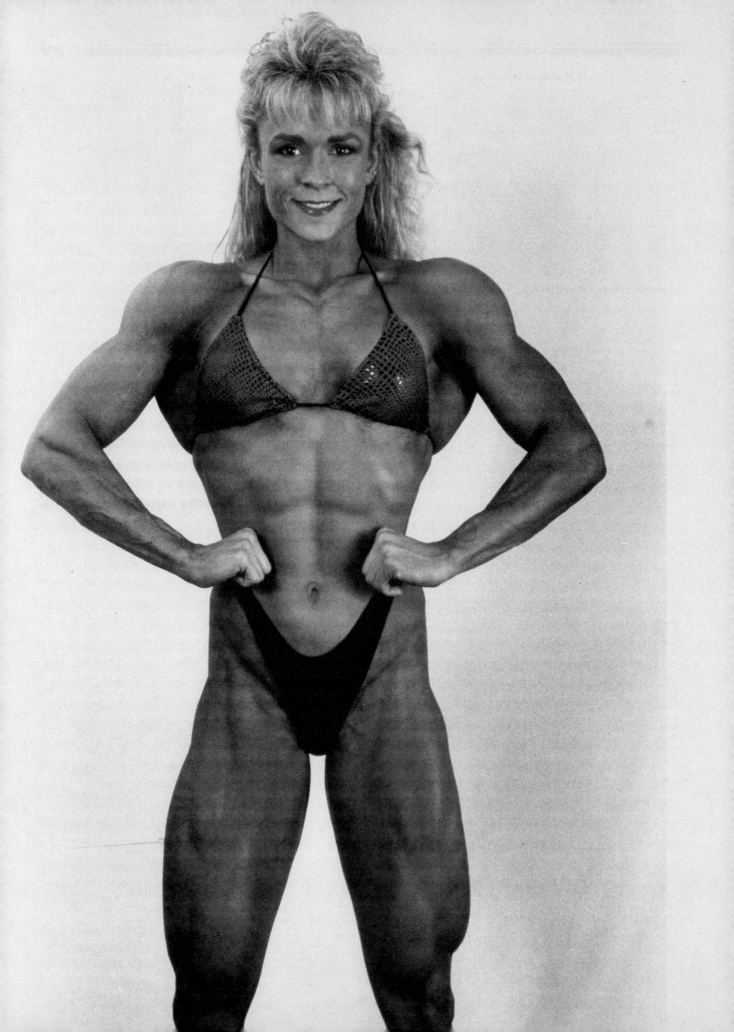

FOUR

SUPPLEMENTATION: THE EXTRA EDGE

Your ability to build muscle is largely set by the amount of calories and nutrients you take in. By upping your calories and taking nutritional supplements, you can increase nutrients at the cellular level, and these nutrients supply the building blocks to support muscular growth. For this reason, supplements play a key role in bodybuilding nutrition. In addition to increased growth, they provide many other important benefits when used with proper nutrition.

Supplements, however, are not magic pills and powders that work all by themselves. For supplements to be effective, they must be used in conjunction with proper nutrition—and taken at the proper times and in the right combinations. In fact, don't even consider taking supplements until you are eating properly and taking in enough quality calories. Only when your nutrition program is well established is it time to start a supplement program.

Tonya Knight has it all: muscle, symmetry, and charisma. Photo by Jimmie D. King.

YOUR PERSONAL SUPPLEMENT PROGRAM

The shelves of health food stores are crammed with bottles and jars of supplements, while the pages of bodybuilding magazines are full of all the latest products, many with some very tempting claims. Undeniably, there are plenty of supplements out there, and this array can be confusing. What should you take? What works and what doesn't? What's truth and what's hype?

My approach to supplementation is based on years of experimentation and one-on-one work with the world's top bodybuilders. Over the past 20 years, I have evaluated what certain nutrients can do, and through trial and error, I have determined how supplemental nutrients should be taken for maximum results. In my estimation, there are certain nutritional supplements that uniquely meet the needs of bodybuilders and athletes, and these include: multi-vitamins, multi-mineral-electrolytes, lipotropics, desiccated liver tablets, amino acids (including branched chain aminos and growth-hormone releasers), endurance supplements, carbohydrate supplements, a quality protein powder or protein/carbohydrate bar, and medium-chain fatty acids (MCFAs).

Vitamins

Vitamins are important regulators of metabolism that serve as catalysts in the conversion of food into energy. The following chart identifies the major vitamins and their role in bodybuilding:

Vitamins	Bodybuilding-Related Functions
Vitamin A	Growth and repair; maintenance of healthy skin tissue.
Vitamin B-Complex	Proper metabolism of protein, carbohydrates, and fats; energy production.
Vitamin C	Proper metabolism of fats; formation of certain hormones secreted during exercise and stress; synthesis of collagen (a protein constituent of connective tissue); transportation, absorption, and storage of iron (non-heme iron) obtained from plant sources.
Vitamin D	Normal bone growth and development.
Vitamin E	Protection of cell membranes against oxidative damage associated with exercise; cellular respiration.

Minerals

Your body requires minerals for many processes, including growth and development, metabolism, nerve transmission, muscular contraction, and the formation of bone and tissue. This chart lists the minerals needed for good health, along with their roles in bodybuilding.

Minerals	Bodybuilding-Related Functions
Calcium	Formation of body structures; prevention of bone loss.
Phosphorous	Growth, maintenance, and repair of cells; muscular contraction; energy production.
Magnesium	Protein and carbohydrate metabolism; absorption and metabolism of other minerals; proper functioning of muscles.
Potassium	Muscular contraction; glycogen storage; synthesis of muscular protein from amino acids.
Chloride	Joint and tendon health; distribution of hormones.
Copper	Formation of hemoglobin (an oxygen-carrying protein in the blood) and red blood cells; a constituent of enzymes involved in the breakdown and synthesis of body tissue.
Iodine	Regulation of energy and metabolism.
Iron	Transport of oxygen to tissues for energy.
Boron	Possible elevation of testosterone levels; prevention of bone loss.
Chromium	Normal blood sugar metabolism; possible involvement in the promotion of lean mass.
Manganese	Fatty-acid synthesis; protein, carbohydrate, and fat production; structure of cell mitochondria; prevention of bone loss.
Selenium	Protection of tissues against oxidative damage.
Zinc	Protein, carbohydrate, and fat metabolism; cellular growth and tissue repair; production of hemoglobin; insulin secretion.

Electrolytes

For optimum health, a constant balance must be maintained in the fluid levels of the body, both inside and outside the cells. Fluids protect internal organs, supply nutrients and oxygen to cells and tissues for growth and repair, and transport carbon dioxide and other waste products away from cells.

Ron Love, a former Detroit police officer, is a top Mr. Olympia contender. Photo by J. M. Manion.

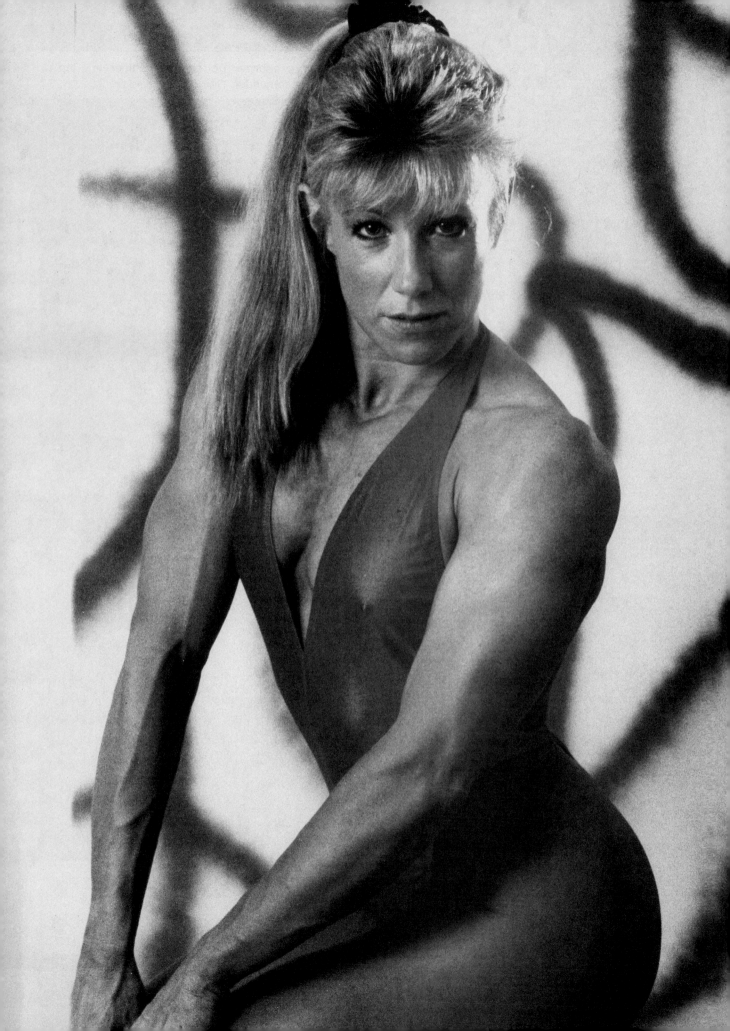

In maintaining this important fluid balance, the presence of certain minerals called electrolytes is vital. The main electrolytes in extra-cellular fluid are sodium, calcium, and chloride, while in the intracellular fluid, the electrolytes are potassium, magnesium, and phosphorous. These nutrients provide a life-sustaining environment for all body cells and must be kept in proper balance.

Hard, intense training can remove needed electrolytes from the body through perspiration. These must be replenished by diet and supplementation if the body is to function at peak levels.

The electrolyte magnesium depends on the presence of calcium for its action. So when selecting a mineral-electrolyte supplement, make sure that the magnesium is equal to or at least 70 percent of the calcium. Additionally, choose mineral-electrolyte supplements which are "chelated." Chelation is a process that binds the mineral to a protein for better absorbability through the small intestine.

Lipotropics

Also known as "fat-burners," lipotropics are nutrients that help your body mobilize and metabolize fat. Typically, these nutrients are found in a single formulation and include the following:

• Inositol. A member of the B-complex vitamin family, inositol stimulates the production of lecithin, a constituent of cells that helps break down cholesterol in the body.

• Choline. This nutrient is another one of the B-complex vitamins. Choline helps prevent the buildup of fat in the liver and helps move fat into cells to be burned for energy. Additionally, choline is involved in the metabolism of nutrients needed for building muscle tissue.

• Betaine. This is a product from the oxidation of choline that is involved in metabolism.

• Methionine. An essential amino acid, methionine helps synthesize choline and is involved in the release of growth hormone in the body. The combination of inositol, choline, betaine, and methionine helps your body mobilize stored fat so that it can be burned for energy.

• L-carnitine. This is a vitamin-like nutrient that is necessary for the utilization of fats by the body, thus sparing carbohydrates and proteins from being used as energy. Even though your body produces carnitine naturally, supplementation can provide extra insurance that adequate levels are maintained in the system.

Desiccated Liver Tablets

Desiccated liver tablets are a concentrated source of liver which has been processed to remove all the fat. This supplement is rich in protein, B-complex vitamins, minerals, and heme iron. Well-absorbed by the body, heme iron is used to manufacture hemoglobin, which builds red blood cells and transports oxygen from the lungs throughout the body.

Amino Acids

Amino acids are the building blocks of protein. Without amino acids, the body cannot manufacture protein, and protein is needed to make muscle. Amino acid supplementation is used to provide an additional source of protein—beyond food—that can be used by the muscles for

A Masters competitor, Kathi Harrison is an inspiration. She has won several championships, including the WNBF (World Natural Bodybuilding Federation) Pro All America and the Pro WNBF World Championship. Photo by Jimmie D. King.

growth and repair. A good base formulation will include the following amino acids:

Amino Acids	Major Functions
L-alanine	Energy production and regulation of blood sugar.
L-aspartic acid	Energy production.
L-cysteine	Protein metabolism.
L-arginine	Growth hormone release (with l-lysine).
L-glutamine	Energy production (with B-complex vitamins B-6, B-3, and magnesium).
L-histidine	Protein synthesis.
L-lysine	Growth hormone release (with l-arginine).
L-methionine	Choline synthesis.
L-phenylalanine	Collagen formation; alertness.
L-proline	Collagen formation.
L-serine	Production of cellular energy.
L-threonine	Energy production.
L-tyrosine	A precursor of adrenaline and thyroid hormones.

Branched-Chain Amino Acids

About 35 percent of your muscles are made up of l-leucine, l-isoleucine, and l-valine, known as the branched-chain amino acids (BCAAs). All three of these nutrients are involved directly in the building of muscle, and deficiencies can lead to muscle loss.

Following a high-protein meal, BCAAs are rapidly absorbed, processed by the liver, and released into the bloodstream. From there, they are taken up by the muscles to be metabolized—unlike other amino acids, which are metabolized in the liver.

BCAAs need insulin to be transported into the muscles for growth and repair. BCAAs, therefore, should always be taken with meals and never on an empty stomach.

Supplemental-Growth Hormone (GH) Releasers

"GH releasers" are another popular amino-acid formulation among body-builders, particularly because they are thought to burn fat and build muscle. There are many types of GH releasers, including the amino acids arginine, lysine, ornithine, tyrosine, and glycine. These nutrients appear to have a stimulatory effect on the production of growth hormone in the body.

Stored in the pituitary gland, growth hormone is involved in the growth of body tissues and has several important effects on the metabolism of protein, carbohydrates, and fats. In protein metabolism, for example, it helps transport amino acids across cellular membranes, increasing the concentration inside cells so that protein synthesis can proceed. Additionally, growth hormone prevents the breakdown of protein and its utilization for energy. Most likely, this occurs because growth hormone can mobilize fat for energy, thus sparing protein.

Growth hormone has a carbohydrate-sparing effect as well because it decreases cellular utilization of glucose. In the tissues, growth hormone also converts fatty acids to acetyl-Co-A, a molecule used in the production of energy.

Growth hormone is secreted throughout a person's lifetime. The rate of secretion can be affected by a number of factors, including nutritional status, exercise (working out does increase the secretion rate somewhat), time of day, and stress.

When given intravenously, certain amino acids seem to trigger the release of growth hormone in the body. The combi-

Roger Stewart's good looks and great physique make him a popular bodybuilder. Photo by J. M. Manion.

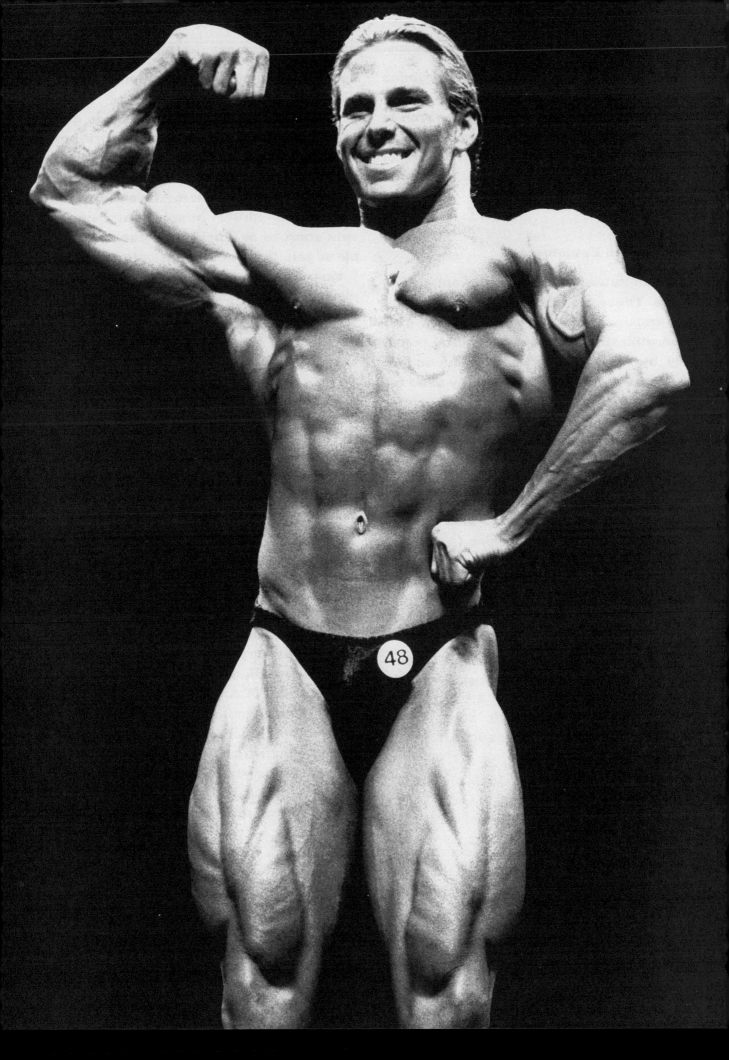

nation of two amino acids—arginine pyroglutamate and lysine monohydrochloride—has been shown in research to be the only oral pair of amino acids to effectively elevate the body's levels of growth hormone. This combination is available in supplement form.

Endurance Enhancers

Certain nutrients appear to affect endurance. These include the following:

• Inosine. This nutrient improves oxygen utilization for better stamina, possibly by forcing additional production of ATP, the direct source of energy used for all physiological processes.

• L-phenylalanine. This is an essential amino acid that acts as a potent mental stimulant for improved concentration during workouts.

• D-phenylalanine. The mirror image of L-phenylalanine, this amino acid inhibits the breakdown of endorphins (a protein-like substance with analgesic properties) for a higher pain threshold.

• Ferulic acid (FRAC). This nutrient stimulates the endocrine system to aid recovery and boost workout capacity.

• Magnesium and potassium aspartates. Hard training produces certain waste products, including ammonia. By turning ammonia into uric acid, aspartates help filter waste products from the system.

Carbohydrate Supplements

For energy to train, your body draws upon glucose stored as glycogen in the muscles. These glycogen reserves are gradually emptied the longer and harder you train, and the result is muscular fatigue. One way to prevent the onset of fatigue and help extend energy is to use a pow-dered carbohydrate supplement in your diet.

Select a formulation that contains glucose polymers, either maltodextrin or rice dextrin. These are slow-releasing carbohydrates derived from grains that provide sustained energy levels. Do not use carbohydrate supplements made with sucrose or fructose. These are simple sugars that convert easily to body fat.

Mixed with water, a carbohydrate supplement can be taken with meals to increase calories, during workouts for extra stamina and energy, and after workouts to initiate recovery.

Protein Powders

Protein powders have been a bodybuilding staple for decades. They provide an additional source of dietary protein, nutrients, and calories. As with all nutritional supplements, you must be selective—and label-conscious—when purchasing a protein powder. The reason is, many protein powders are loaded with fillers and simple sugars, and I have seen athletes gain body fat by using them.

A good protein powder may be enhanced with crystalline free-form amino acids, including the branched-chain amino acids (BCAAs), and two high-quality proteins called calcium caseinate and lactalbumin. A carbohydrate source such as maltodextrin or rice dextrin should be a part of the formulation. These help stimulate the release of insulin, which is required for the transport of BCAAs into the muscles for growth and repair.

Mixed with water or stirred into hot cereal, protein powder should be taken after workouts to supply the nutrients required for recovery and as needed to increase your daily calorie or protein levels. Protein/carbohydrate supplements are also available in bar form.

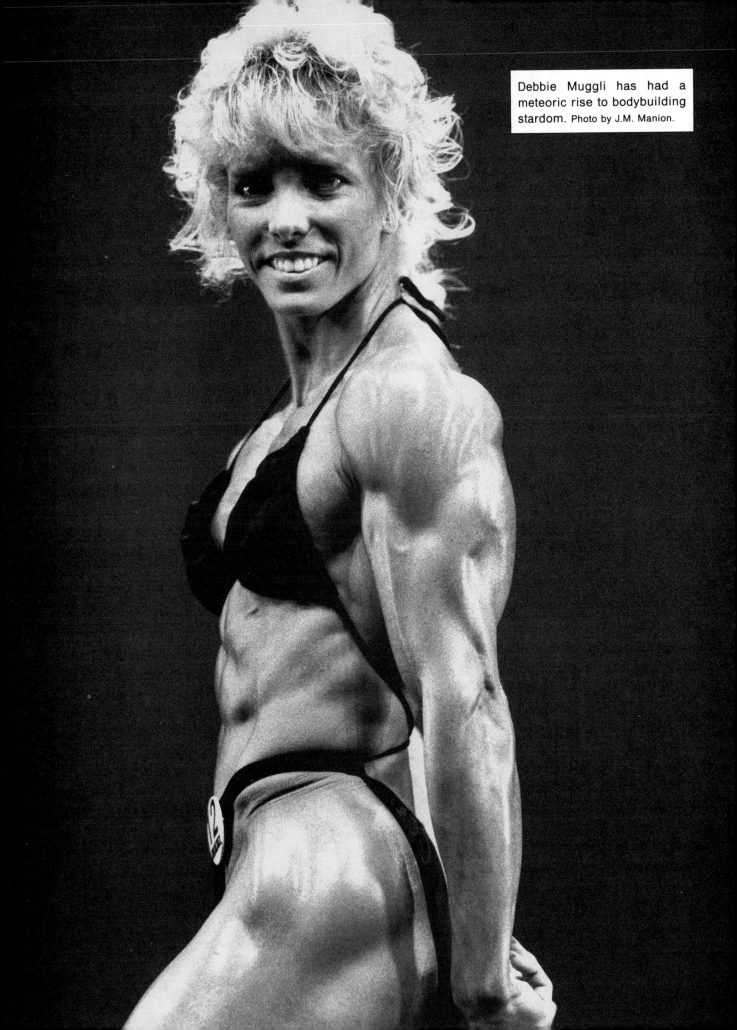

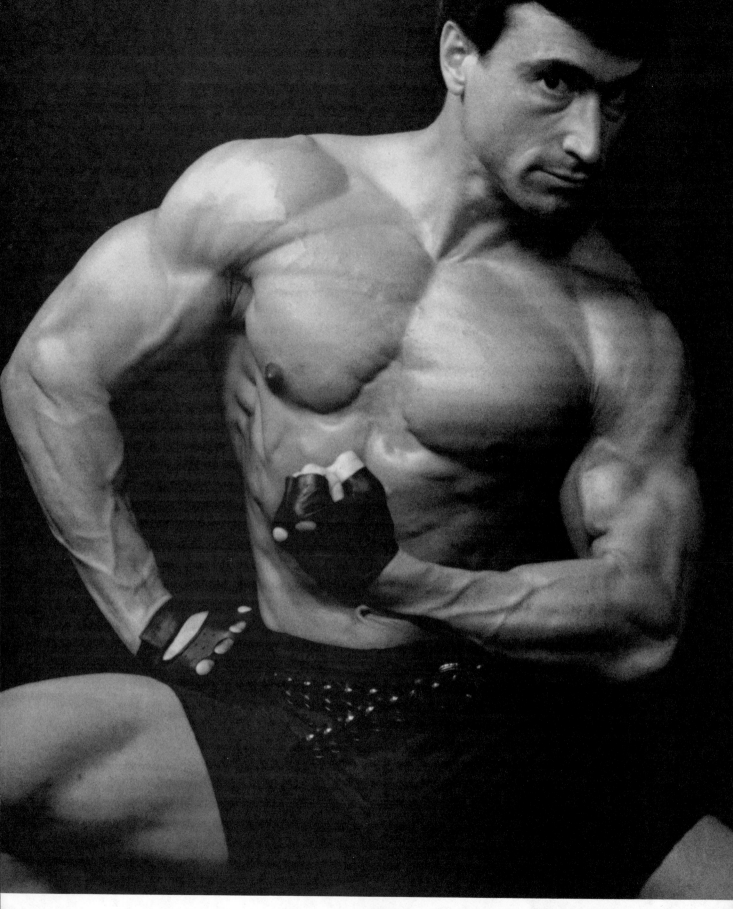

Physique Artist Extraordinaire Russ Testo gives the most entertaining posing routines by combining mime, robotics, acting, dance, and muscle. Photo by J. C. Musco-Studio 59.

Supplementation for Hyper-Recovery

Added to proper nutrition, supplements can help you achieve what I call "hyper-recovery." This refers to the ability to extend your energy and endurance and boost your recuperative powers so that you can train at full capacity and then recover completely from those workouts.

To do that, you should supplement your diet at specific times during the day. For example:

Upon Rising: Take two to three GH releasers on an empty stomach. The morning is one of the periods during the day at which natural levels of growth hormone are thought to be the highest.

With Meals: Because your metabolism is constantly at work, continue to take supplements throughout the day—and always with meals. Their value is increased when you spread them out into equal portions throughout the day. If you take your supplements only in the morning and work out in the afternoon, then very few supplemental nutrients remain for use by the body during training. As your body digests nutrients from food and supplements through the day, messages from the digestive process are relayed throughout the body, signaling your cells to use these nutrients for growth and repair. The supplements you should take with your meals include vitamins (one per meal), minerals and electrolytes (one to two per meal), liver tablets (five or more per meal), amino acids (two or more per meal), lipotropics (one per meal), and supplemental protein in the form of a powder or bar.*

Pre-workout: About 30 minutes to an hour before training, take five endurance-enhancing supplements, one that contains magnesium and potassium aspartates. In preparation for training, take two supplemental GH releasers.

During Workouts: For even greater energy and endurance, sip a carbohydrate beverage during your workouts. This provides a source of carbohydrate other than muscle glycogen. With glycogen spared, fatigue is delayed. Make sure the carbohydrate beverage contains the slow-release carbs maltodextrin or rice dextrin and is free of simple sugars such as fructose and glucose.

Post-training: Muscles are most receptive to synthesizing new glycogen with the first few hours after exercise. To initiate recovery and restore glycogen, take a liquid protein/carbohydrate beverage at this time. Also, take the same supplements you ingest with your meals. That way, you immediately start replacing the nutrients your body has used during training.

Before Bedtime: Take two GH releasers again (on an empty stomach).

Too many bodybuilders make the mistake of trying to train harder—but without the proper nutritional support. This can lead to poor recovery, which is simply undernourishment. Poor nutrition impedes your ability to have productive workouts and to develop new muscle. The harder you train, the more nutrients you will require in order to recover from your workouts and build more muscle. Match your nutrition to your training, and the more intense and effective your workouts will be.

There's one more supplement left to discuss, and that's medium-chain fatty-acid (MCFA) oil. I feel that this supplement is so important to bodybuilders and athletes that it deserves its own chapter.

---

*Certain supplements, including vitamins and minerals, are toxic when taken in high doses. Be sure to use supplements that are formulated to be taken in divided doses throughout the day. Always consult your physician before taking any nutritional supplements.

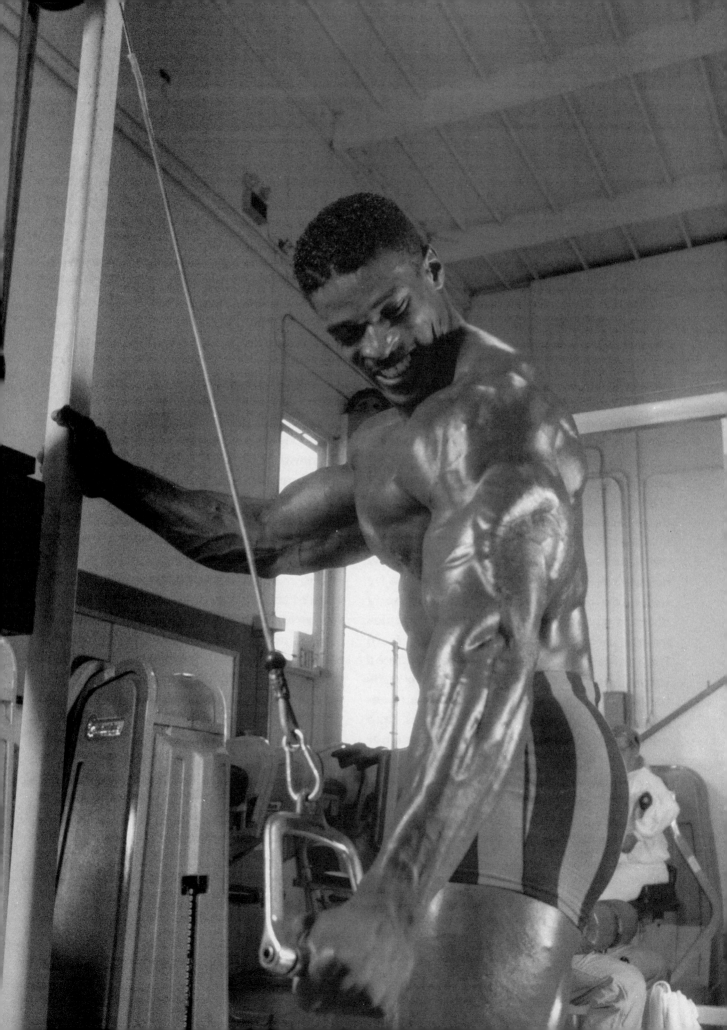

FIVE

MEDIUM-CHAIN FATTY ACIDS: THE PERFECT TRAINING FUEL

Suppose there were a natural food supplement that could supply additional calories to support muscular gains and energy needs—without being stored as body fat. Wouldn't you want such a supplement in your bodybuilding diet?

You bet. There is a supplement with these properties, and it's called a medium-chain fatty acid (MCFA). A key component of my nutrition program, MCFAs are a type of medium-chain triglyceride or MCT oil, a supplement first introduced in 1950 for the treatment of patients with problems absorbing conventional fats. Since then, MCT oil has been used in hospital feeding programs and is now sold in health food stores as a performance-enhancing supplement for athletes, bodybuilders, and other active people.

MCFAs are lipids, refined from coconut oil through a special extraction process. Despite being a coconut-oil derivative, MCFAs are cholesterol free, without any

Ronnie Coleman knows the importance of using MCFA oil to supplement his diet. Photo by Jim Amentler.

of the adverse qualities associated with tropical oils. The molecular structure of MCFAs is quite different from conventional fats such as margarine, butter, and vegetable oils, giving them some very unique properties.

FAT METABOLISM

Understanding the differences between MCFAs and other fats requires a closer look at fats and their function in the body. Conventional fat and body fat are referred to as "long-chain triglycerides" (LCTs) because they are constructed of long fatty-acid groups of 12 or more carbon atoms. MCFAs, on the other hand, contain fatty-acid groups with chains of 6, 8, or 10 carbon atoms—a shorter molecular structure that causes them to be metabolized in an entirely different manner than conventional fats are metabolized.

Before being used for energy, conventional fats (LCTs) must go through an elaborate and slow-moving process in the body. Like most oily substances, LCTs are not very water soluble. In the small intestine, therefore, they must be dissolved by enzymes and bile acids into tiny fat droplets. Cells in the intestinal walls wrap the droplets in special protein blankets so that they can be transported to the lymphatic system (a special type of circulatory system for fluids and fats), which later joins the bloodstream. From there, the fat goes to the liver for further breakdown. Next, it reenters the bloodstream, where it can either be burned as fuel or stored as body fat in fat cells.

The mobilization of fat from storage sites in the body is even more complicated. Stored fat must exit the fat cell, travel through the bloodstream, and enter the liver, and get converted back to a fatty acid. It then reenters the bloodstream to eventually undergo the various chemical reactions involved in energy production.

MCFAs do not require such a complicated digestive process. Because they are more water-soluble than LCTs, MCFAs can be absorbed intact. Nor do they need to be dissolved by enzymes or wrapped in protein blankets. They are transported directly to the liver by the portal vein, completely bypassing the lymphatic system.

When you understand what happens to fats in the liver at the cellular level, you'll understand why MCFAs have very little tendency to be stored as body fat—a property that makes this supplement ideal for bodybuilders and athletes.

Fat-Burning at the Cellular Level

MCFAs are treated differently than LCTs at the cellular level in the liver, the primary site of metabolism. Once inside the cell, fat molecules are burned in cellular furnaces called mitochondria. For LCTs to enter the mitochondria, they require a special transport system called the "carnitine shuttle." When carbohydrates are being burned in the mitochondria, however, LCTs can't get in. The reason is, carbohydrate metabolism creates a by-product that inhibits the carnitine shuttle. As a result, LCTs can be burned only after carbohydrate fuels have been depleted, and this is one reason why conventional fat tends to be stored so easily rather than being used for energy.

By contrast, MCFAs, with their shorter molecular chain, can diffuse through the mitochondrial wall and into the mitochondria, without being ushered in by the carnitine shuttle. Inside the mitochondria, MCFAs are burned for energy—even in the presence of carbohydrates. This is one of the reasons MCFAs are rarely stored as body fat, unlike LCTs.

Burned with carbohydrates, MCFAs help the carbohydrate fuel last longer, thus producing a carbohydrate-sparing effect. The more carbohydrate fuel you have available, the harder you can train. By supplementing your diet with MCFAs, you can spare carbohydrates for longer, more intense workouts.

MCFAs and Muscular Energy

When fats and other nutrients are burned inside the mitochondria, the energy given off is captured by a molecule called ATP. ATP is the direct source of energy used for all body functions, including muscular contraction.

As fat is burned, a compound called acetyl-CoA is produced. It enters a series of chemical reactions known as the Krebs Cycle, which ultimately generates ATP. MCFAs are burned so quickly inside the mitochondria that an enormous amount of acetyl-CoA is produced, and the Krebs Cycle can't handle it all. As a result, some of the acetyl-CoA is converted into ketones, which are by-products of fat metabolism.

This process can occur with conventional fats too. In fact, your body produces ketones from your own body fat during fasting conditions. Under normal circumstances, however, LCTs do not produce ketones because they are not burned as rapidly as MCFAs.

Ketones are released into the bloodstream and are taken up by the muscles to be used for energy. Inside the muscle cells, the ketones are reconverted into acetyl-CoA and further metabolized in the Krebs Cycle to generate ATP.

The Thermic Effect of MCFAs

The process of burning food releases energy. Some of this energy is captured by the body to be used for growth and activity, and some of it is liberated as body heat. As mentioned earlier, the production of heat from the burning of foods is called thermogenesis. Different foods liberate different amounts of heat in the body, and these differences are used to describe what is known as the thermic effect of food (TEF).

The TEF indicates how much of the food is either burned for energy or converted to body weight (muscle or fat). When a food is fully burned, carbon dioxide and water are produced, and these are not stored. Some foods are only partially burned because they supply nutrients for growth and maintenance or because the body easily stores them as body fat. The faster a food burns, the higher its TEF. By eating fast-burning foods and avoiding foods that are easily stored, you tend to stay leaner.

Thermogenesis is related to metabolic rate. After a meal, your metabolic rate increases because food stimulates thermogenesis. Foods with a high TEF tend to elevate the metabolic rate more than foods with a lower TEF.

MCFAs have a very high thermic effect because they are rapidly and efficiently burned, with little tendency to be retained by the body. In one study of the thermic effects of MCFAs and LCTs, ingestion of MCFAs was shown to increase the metabolic rate 12 percent over six hours, compared to only 4 percent over the same period with LCTs.[*] The high TEF of MCFAs is the single most important reason why MCFA calories are rarely stored as body fat.

You can use this information in two ways. First, because your metabolism speeds up after each meal due to thermogenesis, eating frequent meals keeps your metabolic rate high throughout the day. Second, supplementing your diet with MCFAs, with their high TEF, further increases the metabolic rate following meals. To help build your metabolism, it certainly makes sense to eat five to six meals a day and supplement with MCFAs.

Fat-Burning

The restriction of carbohydrates in the diet encourages the body to burn fat for energy. In the absence of carbohydrates, the body releases glucagon (a hormone that opposes the action of insulin) as a signal to mobilize body-fat stores and burn them for energy. When glycogen stores have been depleted, the body starts burning fat for energy.

The problem with restricting carbohydrates, the body's preferred fuel, is the corresponding drop in energy levels. You can, however, use the low-carb strategy

[*]Seaton, T. B., Welle, S. L., Warenko, M. K., and Campbell, R. G. "Thermic Effect of Medium and Long Chain Triglycerides in Man." *The American Journal of Clinical Nutrition* (1986); 44: 630–634.

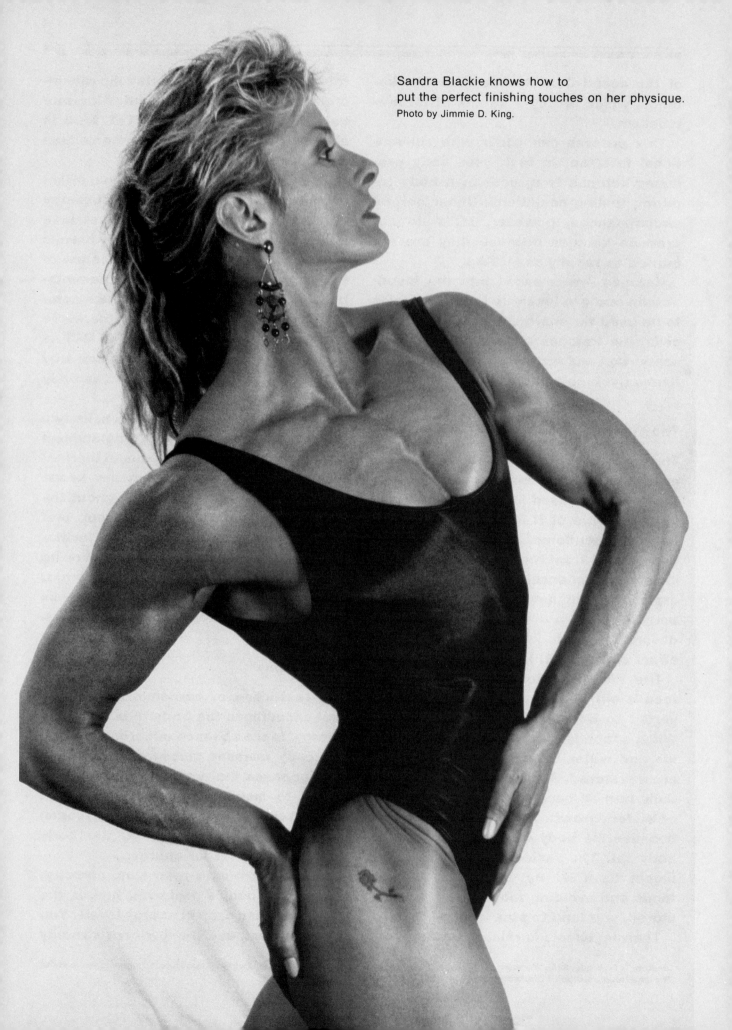

Sandra Blackie knows how to
put the perfect finishing touches on her physique.
Photo by Jimmie D. King.

to shed body fat—but without losing energy. MCFAs are a source of calories your body can use for fuel as a replacement for carbohydrates. By supplementing with MCFAs, you keep your energy levels high, even though you're restricting carbohydrate intake. At the same time, you're creating a dietary and hormonal milieu that is conducive to fat loss. Also, the high thermic effect of MCFAs keeps the metabolic rate elevated. Further details on how to use MCFAs for fat loss are explained in Chapter 7.

Muscularity

Muscular gains result from the increased consumption of quality calories—from food and from supplements—combined with a training program that emphasizes intense exercise, fascial stretching, and aerobics. An excellent way to increase calories and thus promote muscular gain is by supplementing the diet with MCFAs, which supply 114 calories per tablespoon. Providing additional calories is the most important role of MCFAs in building muscle, but the supplement has a secondary role as well.

As mentioned, some MCFAs are turned into ketones during metabolism in the liver, and these can be used by the muscles for energy. The use of ketones spares the burning of branched-chain amino acids in the muscles. With amino acids spared, more protein is available for the muscle repair and growth after training.

How to Take MCFAs

As important as understanding how this supplement works is knowing how to take it correctly. Even though the supplement is a natural product, MCFAs must be gradually introduced into the diet as tolerated and should always be taken with meals. Improper introduction into the diet can cause diarrhea and stomach cramping as a result of the supplement's rapid uptake by the body.

Begin by taking one-half tablespoon with each meal for three days. Then increase that amount to one tablespoon for three more days. Subsequent increases should be made in one-half-tablespoon increments per meal for three days. Higher usage levels depend on your caloric intake and tolerance for MCFAs. If you experience cramping or diarrhea, simply discontinue or decrease your dosage temporarily until your tolerance improves.

You can cook with MCFAs too. Many delicious recipes using this supplement, from chicken ratatouille to sweet-potato oat-bran muffins, are featured in Appendix B.

Because MCFAs contain no essential fatty acids, be sure to take a teaspoon to a tablespoon of EFAs such as flaxseed oil, linseed oil, or safflower oil each day. And, individuals with diabetes, acidosis, or ketosis should consult their physician before using any type of medium-chain fatty-acid oil.

MCFAs split or soften containers and utensils composed of certain plastics, such as polyethlylene and polystyrene. Therefore, the supplement comes in glass bottles and should be used only with glass or metal containers.

By combining MCFAs with the proper diet and exercise program, you'll maximize your results. This amazing lipid, which the medical world has known about for years, supplies the quality calories you need for energy, endurance, and a leaner, more muscular body.

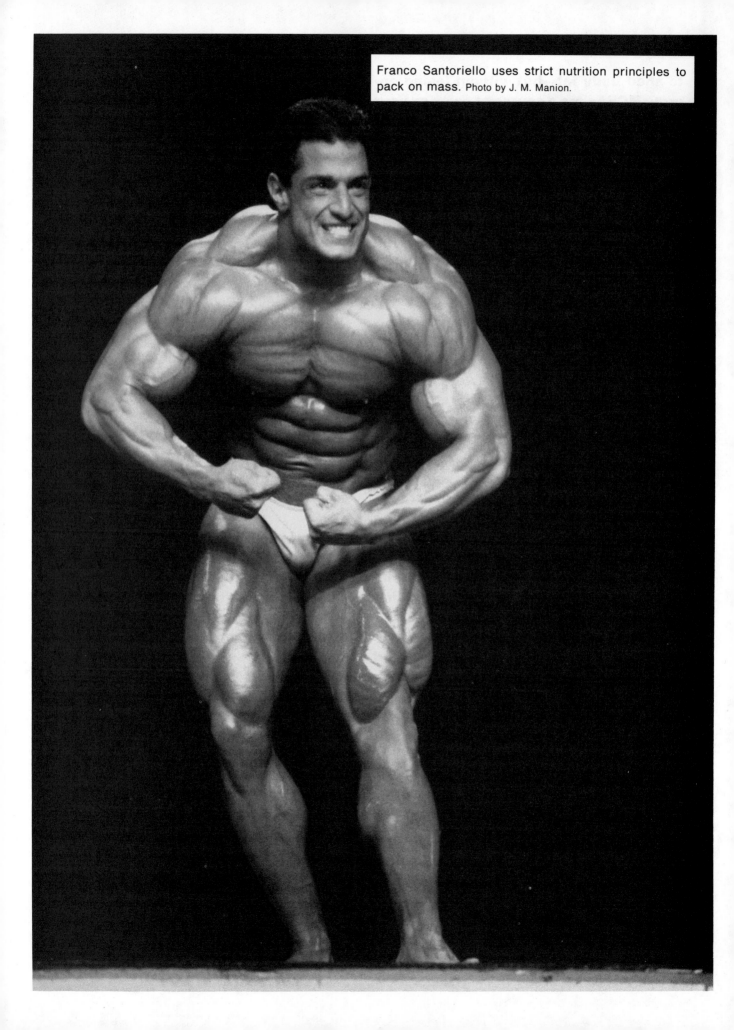

Franco Santoriello uses strict nutrition principles to pack on mass. Photo by J. M. Manion.

SIX

MASS-BUILDING NUTRITION

If your chief goal is to maximize muscular growth, the first step is to gradually increase your calories with the goal of gaining one-half to one pound per 100 pounds of body weight each week. Increase your caloric allotment by 300 to 500 calories every few days until you are gaining at this rate. Because protein is required to construct muscle tissue, be sure you're consuming 1.25 to 1.5 grams of protein daily per pound of body weight. Monitor your progress using my BodyChart System explained in Chapter 11.

You can make muscle only so fast. If you put on weight too rapidly, fat will be gained along with the muscle. Should this happen, decrease your caloric intake by 300 to 500 calories a day. You may also want to slightly reduce your starchy carbohydrate intake and increase your intake of MCFA oil. Eventually, you'll reach a point at which you will gain up to one pound per 100 pounds of body weight each week. Remember, as your body weight increases, you should eat more to support the additional muscle mass and further growth. Each pound of muscle you put on requires another 50 to 100 calories a day.

Here are several sample menus which show how to increase the basic menus by 500 calories.*

2,500 CALORIES

Sample Weight: 135

Time/Food	Amt.	Calories	Protein/g	Fat/g	Carbs/g	Na/mg	K/mg
8 A.M.							
Protein Pwd.	1 Scp.	105	20.0	1.0	6.0	125	50
Corn Grits	50 g.	181	4.4	0.4	39.1	1	40
Egg whites	100 g.	51	10.9	0.0	0.8	146	139
MCFA Oil	0.5 Tbsp.	57					
Subtotal		394	35.3	1.4	45.9	272	229
11 A.M.							
Chicken Breast	100 g.	117	23.4	1.9	0.0	50	320
Potato	75 g.	57	1.6	0.1	51.2	2	264
Asparagus	25 g.	7	0.6	0.1	1.3	1	70
Salad	300 g.	69	3.3	0.3	14.4	48	780
MCFA Oil	1 Tbsp.	114					
Subtotal		364	28.9	2.3	66.8	100	1,434
1 P.M.							
Halibut	125 g.	125	26.1	1.5	0.0	68	561
Brown Rice	50 g.	180	3.8	1.0	38.8	5	107
Corn	25 g.	24	0.9	0.3	5.5	0	70
Green Beans	50 g.	16	1.0	0.1	3.6	4	122
MCFA Oil	0.5 Tbsp.	57					
Subtotal		402	31.7	2.8	47.9	76	860
3 P.M.							
Haddock	125 g.	99	22.9	0.1	0.0	76	380
Black-eyed Peas	100 g.	131	9.0	0.4	23.6	50	387
Broccoli	25 g.	8	0.9	0.1	1.5	4	71
Salad	300 g.	69	3.3	0.3	14.4	48	780
MCFA Oil	1 Tbsp.	114					
Subtotal		421	36.1	0.9	39.5	178	1,618
Carbohydrate Supplement (during and after workout)							
	2 Scps.	210	8.0	0.0	44.0	128	344

*Nutrient values of the menus in this book have been calculated using Parrillo Performance products, including Hi-Protein Powder™, Pro-Carb™, The Bar™, and CapTri®, a medium-chain fatty-acid oil. Other products may yield different calculations.

2,500 CALORIES (Continued)

Time/Food	Amt.	Calories	Protein/g	Fat/g	Carbs/g	Na/mg	K/mg
6 P.M.							
Cod	125 g.	98	22.0	0.4	0.0	89	478
Sweet Potato	100 g.	114	1.7	0.4	26.3	10	243
Cauliflower	25 g.	7	0.7	0.1	1.3	3	74
Lima Beans	25 g.	26	1.6	0.0	4.9	32	123
Salad	300 g.	69	3.3	0.3	14.4	48	780
MCFA Oil	0.5 Tbsp.	57					
Subtotal		370	29.2	1.2	46.9	182	1,697
8 P.M.							
Turkey Breast	100 g.	116	24.6	1.2	0.0	51	320
Potato	100 g.	76	2.1	0.1	68.2	2	352
Zucchini	50 g.	9	0.6	0.1	1.8	1	101
Salad	300 g.	69	3.3	0.3	14.4	48	780
MCFA Oil	0.5 Tbsp.	57					
Subtotal		327	30.6	1.7	84.4	102	1,553
Daily Totals		2,487	199.8	10.2	375.3	1,037	7,734

3,500 CALORIES

Sample Weight: 155

Time/Food	Amt.	Calories	Protein/g	Fat/g	Carbs/g	Na/mg	K/mg
8 A.M.							
Protein Pwd.	1 Scp.	105	20.0	1.0	6.0	125	50
Corn Grits	50 g.	181	4.4	0.4	39.1	1	40
Egg whites	100 g.	51	10.9	0.0	0.8	146	139
MCFA Oil	1 Tbsp.	114					
Subtotal		451	35.3	1.4	45.9	272	229
11 A.M.							
Chicken Breast	150 g.	176	35.1	2.9	0.0	75	480
Potato	125 g.	95	2.6	0.1	85.3	3	440
Asparagus	50 g.	13	1.3	0.1	2.5	1	139
Salad	300 g.	69	3.3	0.3	14.4	48	780
MCFA Oil	1.5 Tbsp.	171					
Subtotal		524	42.3	3.4	102.2	127	1,839
1 P.M.							
Halibut	125 g.	125	26.1	1.5	0.0	68	561
Brown Rice	75 g.	270	5.6	1.4	58.2	7	161
Corn	50 g.	48	1.8	0.5	11.1	0	140
Green Beans	50 g.	16	1.0	0.1	3.6	4	122
MCFA Oil	1.5 Tbsp.	171					
Subtotal		630	34.5	3.5	72.8	78	983
3 P.M.							
Haddock	125 g.	99	22.9	0.1	0.0	76	380
Black-eyed Peas	125 g.	164	11.3	0.5	29.5	63	484
Broccoli	75 g.	24	2.7	0.2	4.4	11	212
Salad	300 g.	69	3.3	0.3	14.4	48	780
MCFA Oil	1.5 Tbsp.	171					
Subtotal		527	40.1	1.2	48.3	198	1,855
Carbohydrate Supplement (during and after workout)							
	3 Scps.	315	12.0	0.0	66.0	192	516
6 P.M.							
Cod	125 g.	98	22.0	0.4	0.0	89	478
Sweet Potato	100 g.	114	1.7	0.4	26.3	10	243
Cauliflower	50 g.	14	1.4	0.1	2.6	7	148
Lima Beans	75 g.	77	4.7	0.1	14.6	97	368
Salad	300 g.	69	3.3	0.3	14.4	48	780
MCFA Oil	1.5 Tbsp.	171					
Subtotal		542	33.0	1.3	57.9	250	2,016
8 P.M.							
Turkey Breast	100 g.	116	24.6	1.2	0.0	51	320
Potato	175 g.	133	3.7	0.2	119.4	4	616
Zucchini	75 g.	13	0.9	0.1	2.7	1	152
Salad	300 g.	69	3.3	0.3	14.4	48	780
MCFA Oil	1.5 Tbsp.	171					
Subtotal		502	32.5	1.8	136.5	103	1,868
Daily Totals		3,489	229.6	12.5	529.5	1,219	9,306

4,500 CALORIES

Sample Weight: 165

Time/Food	Amt.	Calories	Protein/g	Fat/g	Carbs/g	Na/mg	K/mg
8 A.M.							
Protein Pwd.	1 Scp.	105	20.0	1.0	6.0	125	50
Shredded Wheat	100 g.	354	9.9	2.0	79.9	3	348
Egg whites	100 g.	51	10.9	0.0	0.8	146	139
MCFA Oil	2 Tbsp.	228					
Subtotal		738	40.8	3.0	86.7	274	537
11 A.M.							
Chicken Breast	150 g.	176	35.1	2.9	0.0	75	480
Potato	175 g.	133	3.7	0.2	119.4	4	616
Asparagus	75 g.	20	1.9	0.2	3.8	2	209
Salad	300 g.	69	3.3	0.3	14.4	48	780
MCFA Oil	2 Tbsp.	228					
Subtotal		625	44.0	3.5	137.5	128	2,085
1 P.M.							
Halibut	125 g.	125	26.1	1.5	0.0	68	561
Brown Rice	100 g.	360	7.5	1.9	77.6	9	214
Corn	75 g.	72	2.6	0.8	16.6	0	210
Green Beans	75 g.	24	1.4	0.2	5.3	5	182
MCFA Oil	2 Tbsp.	228					
Subtotal		809	37.7	4.3	99.5	82	1,168
3 P.M.							
Haddock	125 g.	99	22.9	0.1	0.0	76	380
Black-eyed Peas	150 g.	197	13.5	0.6	35.4	75	581
Broccoli	100 g.	32	3.6	0.3	5.9	15	282
Salad	300 g.	69	3.3	0.3	14.4	48	780
MCFA Oil	2.5 Tbsp.	285					
Subtotal		681	43.3	1.3	55.7	214	2,023
Carbohydrate Supplement (during and after workout)							
	3 Scps.	315	12.0	0.0	66.0	192	516
6 P.M.							
Cod	125 g.	98	22.0	0.4	0.0	89	478
Sweet Potato	150 g.	171	2.6	0.6	39.5	15	365
Cauliflower	75 g.	20	2.0	0.2	3.9	10	221
Lima Beans	75 g.	77	4.7	0.1	14.6	97	368
Salad	300 g.	69	3.3	0.3	14.4	48	780
MCFA Oil	2 Tbsp.	228					
Subtotal		662	34.5	1.5	72.4	258	2,211
8 P.M.							
Turkey Breast	100 g.	116	24.6	1.2	0.0	51	320
Potato	175 g.	133	3.7	0.2	119.4	4	616
Zucchini	125 g.	21	1.5	0.1	4.5	1	253
Salad	300 g.	69	3.3	0.3	14.4	48	780
MCFA Oil	2.5 Tbsp.	285					
Subtotal		624	33.1	1.8	138.3	104	1969
Daily Totals		4,455	245.3	15.4	656.0	1,252	10,507

5,500 CALORIES

Sample Weight: 180

Time/Food	Amt.	Calories	Protein/g	Fat/g	Carbs/g	Na/mg	K/mg
8 A.M.							
Protein Pwd.	1 Scp.	105	20.0	1.0	6.0	125	50
Oatmeal	100 g.	390	14.2	7.4	68.2	2	352
Egg whites	100 g.	51	10.9	0.0	0.8	146	139
MCFA Oil	3 Tbsp.	342					
Subtotal		888	45.1	8.4	75.0	273	541

Ronnie Coleman trains hard and stays in excellent shape all year. Photo by Jim Amentler.

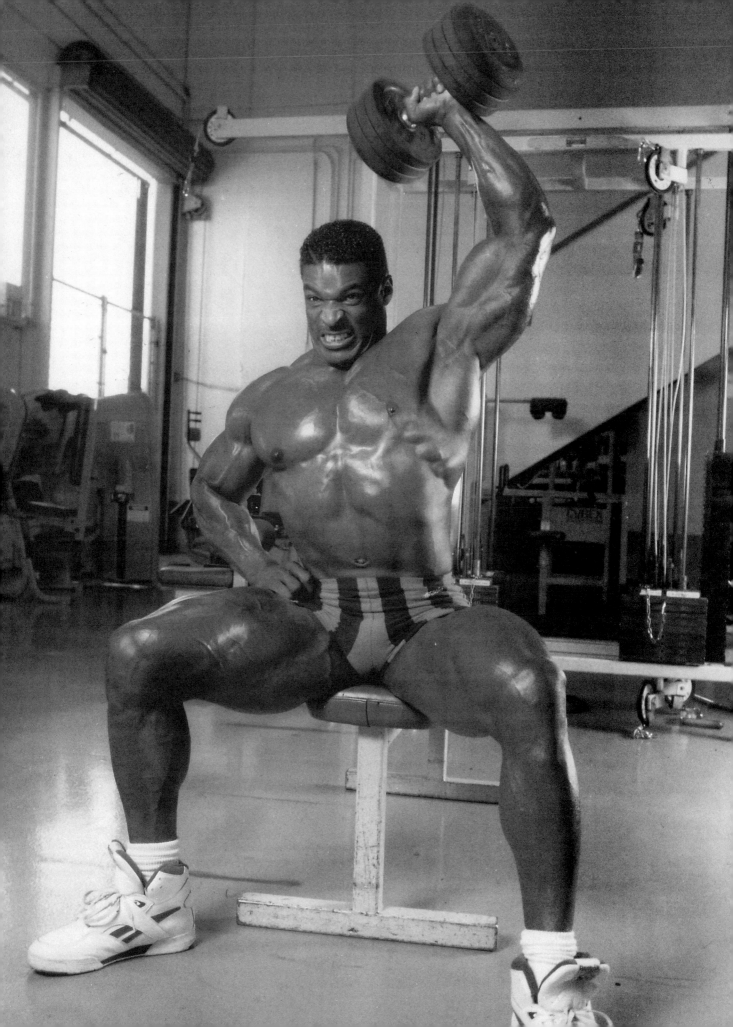

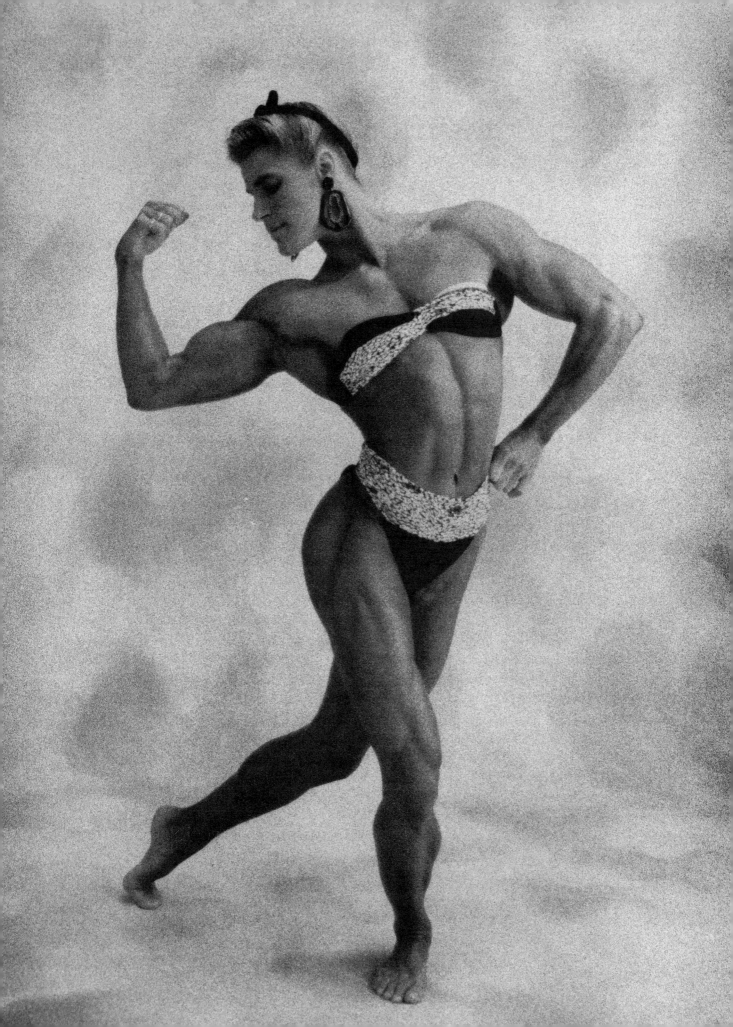

5,500 CALORIES (Continued)

Time/Food	Amt.	Calories	Protein/g	Fat/g	Carbs/g	Na/mg	K/mg
11 A.M.							
Chicken Breast	150 g.	176	35.1	2.9	0.0	75	480
Potato	225 g.	171	4.7	0.2	153.5	5	792
Asparagus	125 g.	33	3.1	0.3	6.3	3	348
Salad	300 g.	69	3.3	0.3	14.4	48	780
MCFA Oil	3 Tbsp.	342					
Subtotal		790	46.3	3.6	174.1	130	2,400
1 P.M.							
Halibut	125 g.	125	26.1	1.5	0.0	68	561
Brown Rice	100 g.	360	7.5	1.9	77.6	9	214
Corn	125 g.	120	4.4	1.3	27.6	0	350
Green Beans	75 g.	24	1.4	0.2	5.3	5	182
MCFA Oil	2.5 Tbsp.	285					
Subtotal		914	39.4	4.8	110.6	82	1,308
3 P.M.							
Haddock	150 g.	119	27.5	0.2	0.0	92	456
Black-eyed Peas	200 g.	262	18.0	0.8	47.2	100	774
Broccoli	125 g.	40	4.5	0.4	7.4	19	353
Salad	300 g.	69	3.3	0.3	14.4	48	780
MCFA Oil	3 Tbsp.	342					
Subtotal		832	53.3	1.6	69.0	258	2,363
Carbohydrate Supplement (during and after workout)							
	4 Scps.	420	16.0	0.0	88.0	256	688
6 P.M.							
Cod	125 g.	98	22.0	0.4	0.0	89	478
Sweet Potato	225 g.	257	3.8	0.9	59.2	23	547
Cauliflower	75 g.	20	2.0	0.2	3.9	10	221
Lima Beans	150 g.	153	9.3	0.2	29.3	194	735
Salad	300 g.	69	3.3	0.3	14.4	48	780
MCFA Oil	3 Tbsp.	342					
Subtotal		938	40.5	1.9	106.7	363	2,761
8 P.M.							
Turkey Breast	100 g.	116	24.6	1.2	0.0	51	320
Potato	200 g.	152	4.2	0.2	136.4	4	704
Zucchini	125 g.	21	1.5	0.1	4.5	1	253
Salad	300 g.	69	3.3	0.3	14.4	48	780
MCFA Oil	3 Tbsp.	342					
Subtotal		700	33.6	1.8	155.3	104	2,057
Daily Totals		5,482	274.1	22.2	778.7	1,466	12,116

6,500 CALORIES

Sample Weight: 192

Time/Food	Amt.	Calories	Protein/g	Fat/g	Carbs/g	Na/mg	K/mg
8 A.M.							
Protein Pwd.	1 Scp.	105	20.0	1.0	6.0	125	50
Corn Grits	100 g.	362	8.7	0.8	78.1	1	80
Egg whites	100 g.	51	10.9	0.0	0.8	146	139
MCFA Oil	3.5 Tbsp.	399					
Subtotal		917	39.6	1.8	84.9	272	269
11 A.M.							
Chicken Breast	150 g.	176	35.1	2.9	0.0	75	480
Potato	250 g.	190	5.3	0.3	170.5	5	880
Asparagus	150 g.	39	3.8	0.3	7.5	3	417
Salad	400 g.	92	4.4	0.4	19.2	64	1,040
MCFA Oil	4 Tbsp.	456					
Subtotal		953	48.5	3.8	197.2	147	2,817

1 P.M.

Time/Food	Amt.	Calories	Protein/g	Fat/g	Carbs/g	Na/mg	K/mg
Halibut	125 g.	125	26.1	1.5	0.0	68	561
Brown Rice	150 g.	540	11.3	2.9	116.4	14	321
Corn	150 g.	144	5.3	1.5	33.2	0	420
Green Beans	125 g.	40	2.4	0.3	8.9	9	304
MCFA Oil	3.5 Tbsp.	399					
Subtotal		1,248	45.0	6.1	158.4	90	1,606
3 P.M.							
Haddock	125 g.	99	22.9	0.1	0.0	76	380
Black-eyed Peas	225 g.	295	20.3	0.9	53.1	113	871
Broccoli	200 g.	64	7.2	0.6	11.8	30	564
Salad	400 g.	92	4.4	0.4	19.2	64	1,040
MCFA Oil	4 Tbsp.	456					
Subtotal		1,006	54.7	2.0	84.1	283	2,855
Carbohydrate Supplement (during and after workout)							
	4 Scps.	420	16.0	0.0	88.0	256	688
6 P.M.							
Cod	125 g.	98	22.0	0.4	0.0	89	478
Sweet Potato	225 g.	257	3.8	0.9	59.2	23	547
Cauliflower	175 g.	47	4.7	0.4	9.1	23	516
Lima Beans	150 g.	153	9.3	0.2	29.3	194	735
Salad	400 g.	92	4.4	0.4	19.2	64	1,040
MCFA Oil	3.5 Tbsp.	399					
Subtotal		1,045	44.3	2.2	116.7	392	3,316
8 P.M.							
Turkey Breast	125 g.	145	30.8	1.5	0.0	64	400
Potato	250 g.	190	5.3	0.3	170.5	5	880
Zucchini	175 g.	30	2.1	0.2	6.3	2	354
Peas	50 g.	37	2.7	0.2	6.4	65	75
MCFA Oil	4 Tbsp.	456					
Subtotal		857	40.8	2.1	183.2	135	1,709
Daily Totals		6,446	288.9	18.0	912.6	1,574	13,259

7,500 CALORIES

Sample Weight: 205

Time/Food	Amt.	Calories	Protein/g	Fat/g	Carbs/g	Na/mg	K/mg
8 A.M.							
Protein Pwd.	1 Scp.	105	20.0	1.0	6.0	125	50
Shredded Wheat	150 g.	531	14.9	3.0	119.9	5	522
Egg whites	100 g.	51	10.9	0.0	0.8	146	139
MCFA Oil	4 Tbsp.	456					
Subtotal		1,143	45.8	4.0	126.7	276	711
11 A.M.							
Chicken Breast	150 g.	176	35.1	2.9	0.0	75	480
Potato	275 g.	209	5.8	0.3	187.6	6	968
Asparagus	200 g.	52	5.0	0.4	10.0	4	556
Salad	400 g.	92	4.4	0.4	19.2	64	1,040
MCFA Oil	5 Tbsp.	570					
Subtotal		1,099	50.3	3.9	216.8	149	3,044
1 P.M.							
Halibut	125 g.	125	26.1	1.5	0.0	68	561
Brown Rice	175 g.	630	13.1	3.3	135.8	16	375
Corn	175 g.	168	6.1	1.8	38.7	0	490
Green Beans	125 g.	40	2.4	0.3	8.9	9	304
MCFA Oil	4 Tbsp.	456					
Subtotal		1,419	47.8	6.8	183.4	92	1,730
3 P.M.							
Haddock	125 g.	99	22.9	0.1	0.0	76	380
Black-eyed Peas	275 g.	360	24.8	1.1	64.9	138	1,064
Broccoli	225 g.	72	8.1	0.7	13.3	34	635
Salad	400 g.	92	4.4	0.4	19.2	64	1,040
MCFA Oil	5 Tbsp.	570					
Subtotal		1,193	60.1	2.3	97.4	312	3,119
Carbohydrate Supplement (during and after workout)							
	4 Scps.	420	16.0	0.0	88.0	256	688

I've always been impressed with Jackie Paisley's symmetry and muscularity. Photo by Paul B. Goode.

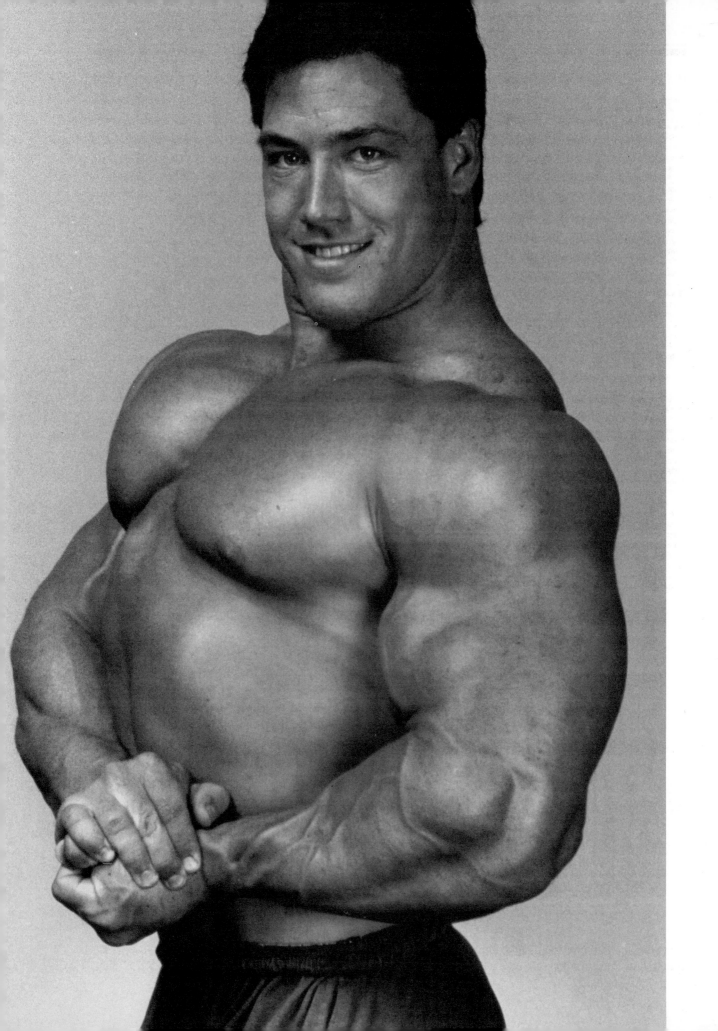

7,500 CALORIES *(Continued)*

Time/Food	Amt.	Calories	Protein/g	Fat/g	Carbs/g	Na/mg	K/mg
6 P.M.							
Cod	125 g.	98	22.0	0.4	0.0	89	478
Sweet Potato	275 g.	314	4.7	1.1	72.3	28	668
Cauliflower	175 g.	47	4.7	0.4	9.1	23	516
Lima Beans	175 g.	179	10.9	0.2	34.1	226	858
Salad	400 g.	92	4.4	0.4	19.2	64	1,040
MCFA Oil	4 Tbsp.	456					
Subtotal		1,185	46.7	2.4	134.8	429	3,560
8 P.M.							
Turkey Breast	125 g.	145	30.8	1.5	0.0	64	400
Potato	275 g.	209	5.8	0.3	187.6	6	968
Zucchini	200 g.	34	2.4	0.2	7.2	2	404
Peas	100 g.	73	5.4	0.3	12.8	129	150
MCFA Oil	5 Tbsp.	570					
Subtotal		1,031	44.3	2.3	207.6	200	1,922
Daily Totals		7,489	310.9	21.7	1,054.4	1,713	14,773

8,500 CALORIES

Sample Weight: 215

Time/Food	Amt.	Calories	Protein/g	Fat/g	Carbs/g	Na/mg	K/mg
8 A.M.							
Protein Pwd.	1 Scp.	105	20.0	1.0	6.0	125	50
Corn Grits	150 g.	543	13.1	1.2	117.2	2	120
Egg whites	100 g.	51	10.9	0.0	0.8	146	139
MCFA Oil	5 Tbsp.	570					
Subtotal		1,269	44.0	2.2	124.0	273	309
11 A.M.							
Chicken Breast	150 g.	176	35.1	2.9	0.0	75	480
Potato	325 g.	247	6.8	0.3	221.7	7	1,144
Asparagus	225 g.	59	5.6	0.5	11.3	5	626
Salad	400 g.	92	4.4	0.4	19.2	64	1,040
MCFA Oil	5 Tbsp.	570					
Subtotal		1,143	52.0	4.0	252.1	150	3,290
1 P.M.							
Halibut	125 g.	125	26.1	1.5	0.0	68	561
Brown Rice	225 g.	810	16.9	4.3	174.6	20	482
Corn	200 g.	192	7.0	2.0	44.2	0	560
Green Beans	125 g.	40	2.4	0.3	8.9	9	304
MCFA Oil	5 Tbsp.	570					
Subtotal		1,737	52.4	8.0	227.7	97	1,907
3 P.M.							
Haddock	125 g.	99	22.9	0.1	0.0	76	380
Black-eyed Peas	300 g.	393	27.0	1.2	70.8	150	1,161
Broccoli	225 g.	72	8.1	0.7	13.3	34	635
Salad	400 g.	92	4.4	0.4	19.2	64	1,040
MCFA Oil	5 Tbsp.	570					
Subtotal		1,226	62.4	2.4	103.3	324	3,216
Carbohydrate Supplement (during and after workout)							
	4 Scps.	420	16.0	0.0	88.0	256	688
6 P.M.							
Cod	125 g.	98	22.0	0.4	0.0	89	478
Sweet Potato	325 g.	371	5.5	1.3	85.5	33	790
Cauliflower	175 g.	47	4.7	0.4	9.1	23	516
Lima Beans	225 g.	230	14.0	0.2	43.9	290	1,103
Salad	400 g.	92	4.4	0.4	19.2	64	1,040
MCFA Oil	5 Tbsp.	570					
Subtotal		1,407	50.6	2.7	157.7	498	3,926

Time/Food	Amt.	Calories	Protein/g	Fat/g	Carbs/g	Na/mg	K/mg
8 P.M.							
Turkey Breast	125 g.	145	30.8	1.5	0.0	64	400
Potato	350 g.	266	7.4	0.4	238.7	7	1,232
Zucchini	200 g.	34	2.4	0.2	7.2	2	404
Peas	125 g.	91	6.8	0.4	16.0	161	188
MCFA Oil	6 Tbsp.	684					
Subtotal		1,220	47.3	2.4	261.9	234	2,224
Daily Totals		8,422	324.5	21.7	1,214.6	1,831	15,558

9,500 CALORIES

Sample Weight: 225

Time/Food	Amt.	Calories	Protein/g	Fat/g	Carbs/g	Na/mg	K/mg
8 A.M.							
Protein Pwd.	1 Scp.	105	20.0	1.0	6.0	125	50
Oatmeal	200 g.	780	28.4	14.8	136.4	4	704
Egg whites	100 g.	51	10.9	0.0	0.8	146	139
MCFA Oil	6 Tbsp.	684					
Subtotal		1,620	59.3	15.8	143.2	275	893
11 A.M.							
Chicken Breast	150 g.	176	35.1	2.9	0.0	75	480
Potato	425 g.	323	8.9	0.4	289.9	9	1,496
Asparagus	225 g.	59	5.6	0.5	11.3	5	626
Salad	400 g.	92	4.4	0.4	19.2	64	1,040
MCFA Oil	6 Tbsp.	684					
Subtotal		1,333	54.1	4.1	320.3	152	3,642
1 P.M.							
Halibut	125 g.	125	26.1	1.5	0.0	68	561
Brown Rice	225 g.	810	16.9	4.3	174.6	20	482
Corn	200 g.	192	7.0	2.0	44.2	0	560
Green Beans	125 g.	40	2.4	0.3	8.9	9	304
MCFA Oil	5 Tbsp.	570					
Subtotal		1,737	52.4	8.0	227.7	97	1,907
3 P.M.							
Haddock	125 g.	99	22.9	0.1	0.0	76	380
Black-eyed Peas	350 g.	459	31.5	1.4	82.6	175	1,355
Broccoli	225 g.	72	8.1	0.7	13.3	34	635
Salad	400 g.	92	4.4	0.4	19.2	64	1,040
MCFA Oil	6 Tbsp.	684					
Subtotal		1,405	66.9	2.6	115.1	349	3,409
Carbohydrate Supplement (during and after workout)							
	4 Scps.	420	16.0	0.0	88.0	256	688
6 P.M.							
Cod	125 g.	98	22.0	0.4	0.0	89	478
Sweet Potato	400 g.	456	6.8	1.6	105.2	40	972
Cauliflower	175 g.	47	4.7	0.4	9.1	23	516
Lima Beans	225 g.	230	14.0	0.2	43.9	290	1,103
Salad	400 g.	92	4.4	0.4	19.2	64	1,040
MCFA Oil	6 Tbsp.	684					
Subtotal		1,606	51.9	3.0	177.4	506	4,108
8 P.M.							
Turkey Breast	125 g.	145	30.8	1.5	0.0	64	400
Potato	450 g.	342	9.5	0.5	306.9	9	1,584
Zucchini	200 g.	34	2.4	0.2	7.2	2	404
Peas	150 g.	110	8.1	0.5	19.2	194	225
MCFA Oil	6 Tbsp.	684					
Subtotal		1,315	50.7	2.6	333.3	268	2,613
Daily Totals		9,436	351.2	36.1	1,404.9	1,903	17,259

Keep your eye on Dennis Newman, the winner of the first Musclemania, sponsored by American Sports Network. Photo by Jimmie D. King.

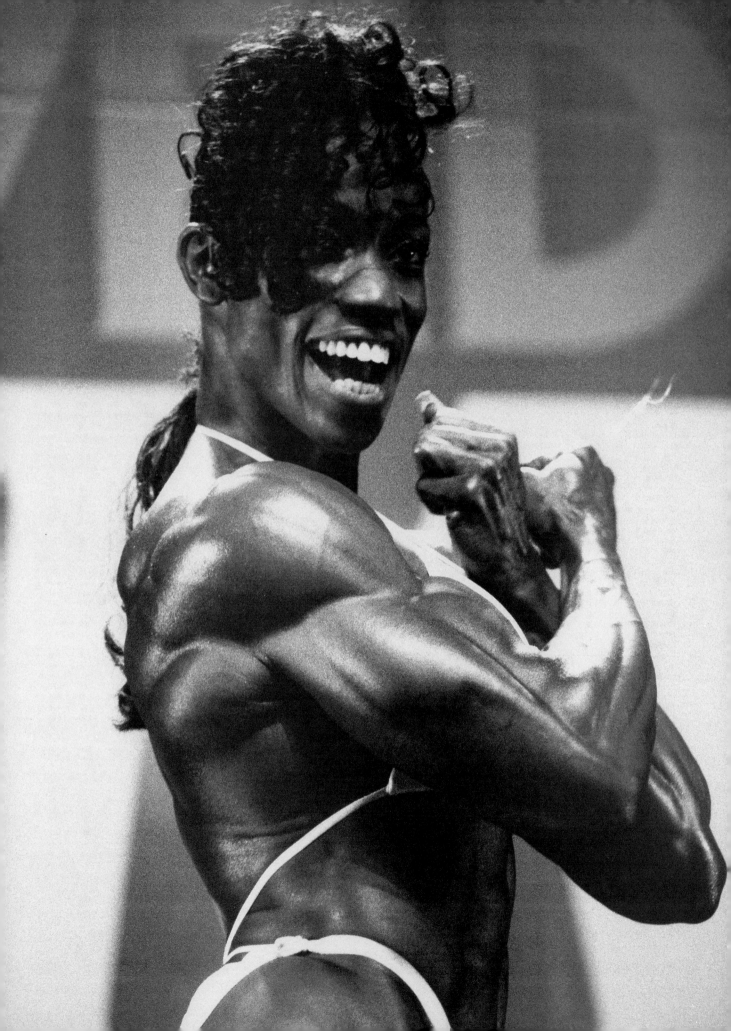

Glycemic Index of Foods

You have probably read or heard about a rating system for foods called the glycemic index. This is a scale developed to rate the body's insulin response to certain foods and is based on a standard of 100, the rating given to glucose when fed orally. Foods with a high glycemic index are typically sugars and refined carbohydrates. Even some starchy carbohydrates have a high glycemic index. Foods high on the scale cause a rapid surge of insulin followed by a plunge of blood sugar that leads to low energy. Foods with a low glycemic index produce a slow, steady release of insulin and yield more sustained energy.

Using the glycemic index to [rate] foods can be misleading—for tw[o rea]sons. First of all, meals do not c[onsist of] single foods. On my nutrition pro[gram, for] example, you eat a specific co[mbination] of foods—a lean protein, one [or two] starchy carbohydrates, and one or tw[o] fibrous vegetables. This combination of foods, specifically the protein with the fiber in the vegetables, slows the digestive process, providing a steady insulin release and therefore lowering the glycemic index of the entire meal. The point is, a single food's rating on the index does not make a major difference as long as it is eaten in slow-release food combinations.

The second problem with this method of rating foods is that some people choose foods low on the index. And many of these foods are simply not good for you, especially if you're trying to gain

mass and [...], for example. [...] index, yet it's full o[...] food with a low g[...] fruit contains [...] erted into a fat b[...] ily stored as bod[...] other hand, ha[...] emic index, yet I [...] dybuilder get fat [...] eep in mind that [...] glycemic index can [...] y fat.

[...] important to understand the effects foods have on [...] e glycemic index does [...] omplete picture. As a [...]g to build lean mass, you [...]ods that are easily stored [...]nd structure your meals to [...]ained energy throughout the

[...]entation

[...]ease your calories to support muscle gains, supplement the nutrition program with MCFA oil, a carbohydrate supplement, and a protein powder or protein/carbohydrate bar. These provide quality calories to your diet without adding fats or simple sugars that easily convert to body fat.

As mentioned, MCFA produces ketones, which can be used by the muscles for fuel just as glycogen is. Ketones are burned preferentially to branched chain amino acids, thereby making more protein available to the muscles for growth and repair.

Use the carbohydrate supplement during workouts for extra energy, after workouts to replenish glycogen stores, and as needed with meals for extra calories. A protein powder or protein/carbohydrate bar should be taken after

Ms. Olympia Lenda Murray always dazzles the fans. Photo by J. M. Manion.

Books are the bees which carry the quickening pollen from one to another mind.
—James Russell Lowell

Penny Price uses stair-climbing equipment to help build cardiovascular density. Photo by Jimmie D. King.

workouts to accelerate recovery and as required to increase your daily calories and protein levels.

Continue taking other supplements, including vitamins, mineral-electrolytes, amino acids, GH releasers, lipotropics, and liver tablets throughout the day, according to the schedule recommended in Chapter 4.

Nutrition for Hard Gainers

Some bodybuilders call themselves "hard gainers," meaning that they have a difficult time putting on muscle mass. Nutrition sets—or extends—the boundaries of how much mass you can gain. If you're a hard gainer, you are simply not eating enough or taking the right nutritional supplements to grow.

To extend your growth potential, you must train your body to process more nutrients by gradually increasing your caloric intake. That way, you build all the systems in your body to use and metabolize food more efficiently, so you become a muscle-building, fat-burning machine.

So-called hard gainers try to increase muscle mass by performing killer workouts. That's fine as long as you are taking in enough nutrients. Unless proper nutrition is in place to help you recover, those workouts will not do any good. Get in the habit of making your nutrition as intense as your training, and your label of "hard gainer" will be a thing of the past.

Cardiovascular Density

Aerobic exercise such as running and cycling is associated primarily with fat-burning. But did you know that it also stimulates muscle growth? The chief reason is that aerobic exercise builds "cardiovascular density," which describes the size and number of blood vessels in your circulatory system.

By forcing oxygen through the body, aerobic exercise increases the size and number of blood vessels. Blood vessels are the "supply routes" that carry oxygen and nutrients to body tissues and remove waste products from tissues. When this circulatory network is expanded, more nutrients can be transported to body tissues, including muscles, to support muscular growth. It's important to note that your muscles are limited in size by the amount of nutrients they can receive. The better your cardiovascular density, the more nutrients there are for your muscles—and the more mass you can gain.

Additionally, aerobic exercise increases your total blood volume, thus enhancing the removal of toxins from your system. You fatigue less easily and recover more quickly.

Getting Ready to "Lean Out"

Many bodybuilders start my program with the objective of losing body fat right away. That's not the optimum approach. Regardless of how much fat you want to lose, you should start the program with the goal of gaining a pound a week at first. That way you can increase muscle (provided you're training, stretching, and doing aerobics), thus boosting your metabolism so you can burn fat much faster. If you try to lose fat first, you won't gain as much muscle. Nor will your metabolism be as efficient.

Once you have put on weight over a period of several weeks, the next step is to lose body fat. And you can do that easily and effectively by following my 12-week, three-stage program, outlined in the next chapter.

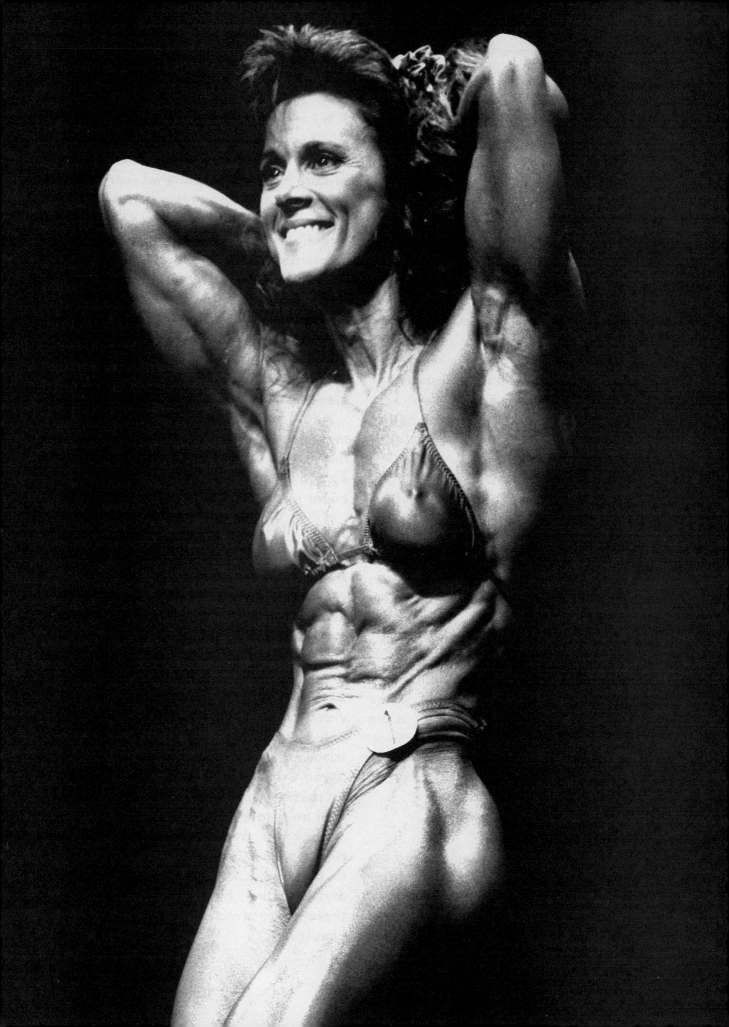

SEVEN

A 12-WEEK FAT-LOSS PROGRAM

Whether you're a competitive bodybuilder preparing for a contest or a bodybuilding enthusiast trying to drop a few pounds, you can do it easily and safely—without sacrificing precious muscle or energy. Best of all, you can do it without making any drastic dietary changes.

To lose body fat, many bodybuilders shift rapidly from normal nutrition right into a near-starvation mode. As noted previously, this deceleration slows your metabolism, making it difficult to burn fat or repair muscle after training. Any drastic reduction in calories causes your body to start feeding on its own muscle tissue, and you lose hard-earned muscle in the process.

My program for losing body fat is a far cry from starvation or drastic caloric restriction. You eat the same healthy foods as previously outlined but in slightly different protein/carbohydrate/fat ratios. By feeding your body instead of starving it, your metabolic rate stays high. That way you burn fat and continue to repair and build muscle. You end up looking harder and more muscular rather than smoother and smaller.

In addition to proper nutrition, another important factor in losing body fat is aerobic exercise, which keeps your metabolism high. When trying to shed body fat, you must increase the time and intensity of your aerobic workouts. I suggest 45 minutes to an hour of aerobics before breakfast, and, if you are preparing for a bodybuilding contest, the same amount in the evening after your last meal.

On my program there are three stages to losing body fat. If you're a competitive bodybuilder, you should follow all three stages, progressing from Stage 1 to Stage 3. Stage 3 is designed to lower your body-fat percentage to contest levels. Men generally compete at 5 percent; women, at about 8 percent. Noncompetitive bodybuilders and athletes interested in getting leaner can simply follow Stage 1 and Stage 2.

Plan to lose no more than one pound of body fat a week. The more slowly you

Janet Tech is a dedicated bodybuilder—and her physique shows it. Photo by J. M. Manion.

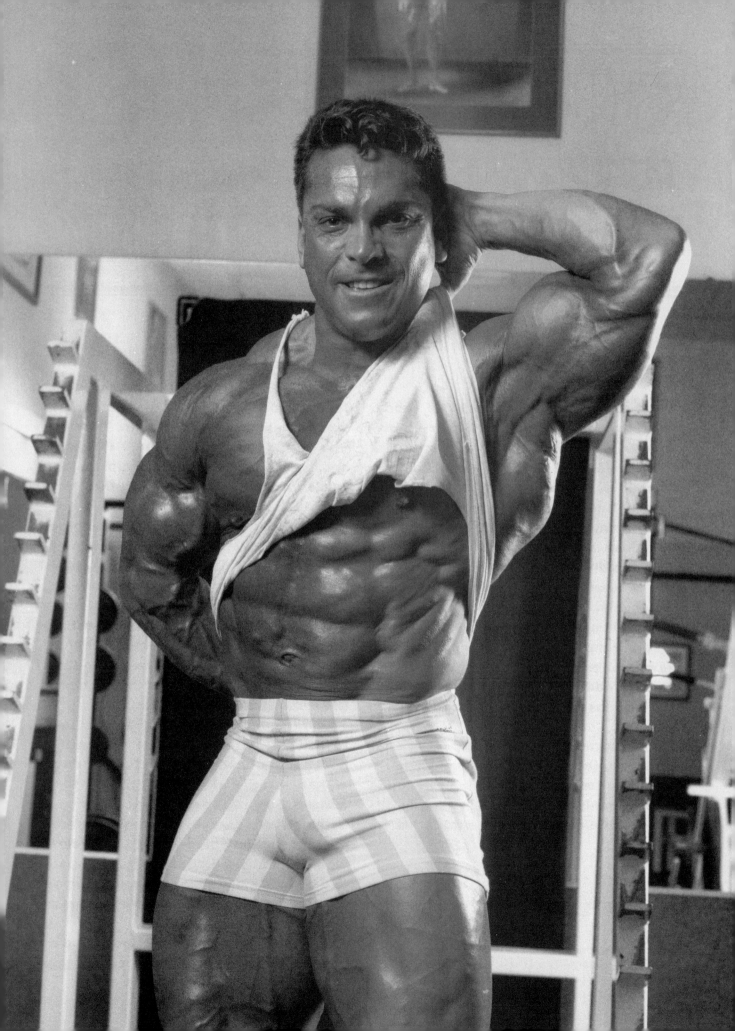

Check out the abs on Rich Gaspari! Photo by Jim Amentler.

shed body fat, the better you'll look and feel. It's important to monitor your ratio of body fat to muscle at least once a week, using my BodyStat Charting System explained in Chapter 11. A scale indicates weight loss, but it can't tell you whether you have lost body fat or muscle. By monitoring your body composition, you'll know when you need to adjust your diet to continue getting lean without losing muscle.

GETTING LEAN: STAGE 1

Stage 1 lasts approximately six weeks. It begins to positively alter your ratio of muscle to body fat and prepares your body for the next two stages. During Stage 1, gradually decrease your intake of starchy carbohydrates to about half and eliminate them from your last meal until you're losing a pound of body fat a week. By reducing carbohydrate intake, you'll have less muscle glycogen left the next morning when you do your aerobic exercise. In this carbohydrate-depleted state, the hormone glucagon is released as a signal for the body to start burning fat. Your body will then start using fatty acids (body fat) for energy, and you'll get leaner as a result.

By lowering your intake of starchy carbohydrates, you also slightly decrease your protein intake because starchy carbohydrates contain some protein. You may want to consume slightly more protein at your last meal. This will also keep you from getting hungry at night. At the same time, eat more fibrous carbohydrates at meals.

Stage 1 is also the time to increase your morning aerobics to an hour. If you're a competitive bodybuilder preparing for a contest, add an additional 45 minutes to an hour of aerobics after your last meal. If you ever feel low on energy as a result of increasing aerobics, add some starchy carbs back into your diet.

To sum up Stage 1:

Reduce your intake of starchy carbohydrates.

Increase your intake of fibrous carbohydrates.

Increase your aerobics.

Stage 1 Menus

Here are sample menus for Stage 1:*

2,000 CALORIES

Time/Food	Amt.	Calories	Protein/g	Fat/g	Carbs/g	Na/mg	K/mg
8 A.M.							
Protein Pwd.	1 Scp.	105	20.0	1.0	6.0	125	50
Oatmeal	25 g.	98	3.6	1.9	17.1	1	88
Egg whites	100 g.	51	10.9	0.0	0.8	146	139
MCFA Oil	0.5 Tbsp.	57					
Subtotal		311	34.5	2.9	23.9	272	277
11 A.M.							
Chicken Breast	75 g.	88	17.6	1.4	0.0	38	240
Potato	25 g.	19	0.5	0.0	17.1	1	88
Asparagus	25 g.	7	0.6	0.1	1.3	1	70
Salad	300 g.	69	3.3	0.3	14.4	48	780
MCFA Oil	1 Tbsp.	114					
Subtotal		296	22.0	1.8	32.7	87	1,178
1 P.M.							
Halibut	100 g.	100	20.9	1.2	0.0	54	449
Corn	50 g.	48	1.8	0.5	11.1	0	140
Green Beans	25 g.	8	0.5	0.1	1.8	2	61
MCFA Oil	0.5 Tbsp.	57					
Subtotal		213	23.1	1.8	12.8	56	650
3 P.M.							
Haddock	125 g.	99	22.9	0.1	0.0	76	380
Black-eyed Peas	25 g.	33	2.3	0.1	5.9	13	97
Broccoli	25 g.	8	0.9	0.1	1.5	4	71
Salad	300 g.	69	3.3	0.3	14.4	48	780
MCFA Oil	1 Tbsp.	114					
Subtotal		323	29.3	0.6	21.8	141	1,327
Carbohydrate Supplement (during and after workout)							
	2 Scps.	210	8.0	0.0	44.0	128	344

*Nutrient values of the menus in this book have been calculated using Parrillo Performance products, including Hi-Protein Powder℗, Pro-Carb℗, The Bar℗, and CapTri®, a medium-chain fatty acid oil. Other products may yield different calculations.

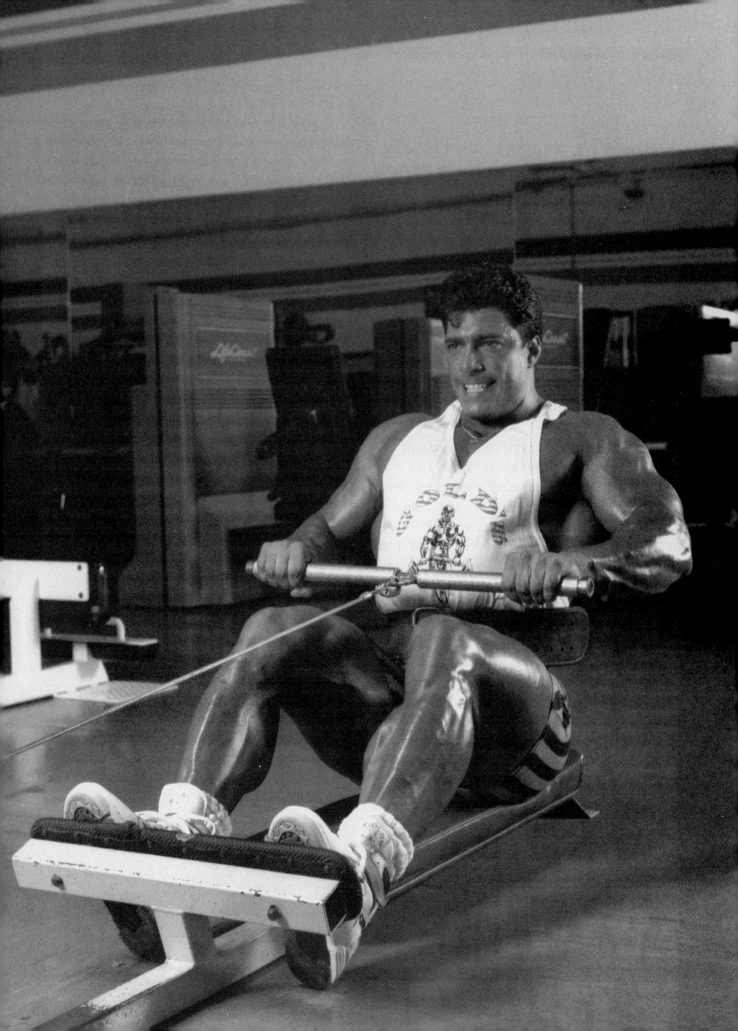

2,000 CALORIES *(Continued)*

Time/Food	Amt.	Calories	Protein/g	Fat/g	Carbs/g	Na/mg	K/mg
6 P.M.							
Cod	50 g.	117	26.4	0.5	0.0	107	573
Sweet Potato	25 g.	29	0.4	0.1	6.6	3	61
Cauliflower	25 g.	7	0.7	0.1	1.3	3	74
Salad	300 g.	69	3.3	0.3	14.4	48	780
MCFA Oil	0.5 Tbsp.	57					
Subtotal		278	30.8	0.9	22.3	160	1,488
8 P.M.							
Turkey Breast	150 g.	174	36.9	1.8	0.0	77	480
Zucchini	25 g.	4	0.3	0.0	0.9	0	51
Salad	300 g.	69	3.3	0.3	14.4	48	780
MCFA Oil	0.5 Tbsp.	57					
Subtotal		304	40.5	2.1	15.3	125	1,311
Daily Totals		1,935	188.2	10.0	172.7	967	6,574

3,000 CALORIES

Time/Food	Amt.	Calories	Protein/g	Fat/g	Carbs/g	Na/mg	K/mg
8 A.M.							
Protein Pwd.	1 Scp.	105	20.0	1.0	6.0	125	50
Oatmeal	50 g.	195	7.1	3.7	34.1	1	176
Egg whites	100 g.	51	10.9	0.0	0.8	146	139
MCFA Oil	2 Tbsp.	228					
Subtotal		579	38.0	4.7	40.9	272	365
11 A.M.							
Chicken Breast	150 g.	176	35.1	2.9	0.0	75	480
Potato	75 g.	57	1.6	0.1	51.2	2	264
Asparagus	50 g.	13	1.3	0.1	2.5	1	139
Salad	300 g.	69	3.3	0.3	14.4	48	780
MCFA Oil	2 Tbsp.	228					
Subtotal		543	41.2	3.3	68.1	126	1,663
1 P.M.							
Halibut	125 g.	125	26.1	1.5	0.0	68	561
Brown Rice	50 g.	180	3.8	1.0	38.8	5	107
Corn	25 g.	24	0.9	0.3	5.5	0	70
Green Beans	75 g.	24	1.4	0.2	5.3	5	182
MCFA Oil	1 Tbsp.	114					
Subtotal		467	32.2	2.9	49.7	77	921
3 P.M.							
Haddock	125 g.	99	22.9	0.1	0.0	76	380
Black-eyed Peas	50 g.	66	4.5	0.2	11.8	25	194
Broccoli	75 g.	24	2.7	0.2	4.4	11	212
Salad	300 g.	69	3.3	0.3	14.4	48	780
MCFA Oil	2 Tbsp.	228					
Subtotal		485	33.4	0.9	30.6	161	1,565
Protein/Carbohydrate Bar (after workout)							
	1 Bar	240	11.0	1.0	38.0	50	210
6 P.M.							
Cod	150 g.	117	26.4	0.5	0.0	107	573
Sweet Potato	50 g.	57	0.9	0.2	13.2	5	122
Cauliflower	50 g.	14	1.4	0.1	2.6	7	148
Lima Beans	25 g.	26	1.6	0.0	4.9	32	123
Salad	300 g.	69	3.3	0.3	14.4	48	780
MCFA Oil	2 Tbsp.	228					
Subtotal		510	33.5	1.1	35.0	198	1,745

Time/Food	Amt.	Calories	Protein/g	Fat/g	Carbs/g	Na/mg	K/mg
8 P.M.							
Turkey Breast	100 g.	116	24.6	1.2	0.0	51	320
Broccoli	75 g.	24	2.7	0.2	4.4	11	212
Zucchini	100 g.	17	1.2	0.1	3.6	1	202
Salad	300 g.	69	3.3	0.3	14.4	48	780
MCFA Oil	2 Tbsp.	228					
Subtotal		454	31.8	1.8	22.4	111	1,514
Daily Totals		3,278	221.0	15.6	284.7	995	7,982

5,000 CALORIES

Time/Food	Amt.	Calories	Protein/g	Fat/g	Carbs/g	Na/mg	K/mg
8 A.M.							
Protein Pwd.	1 Scp.	105	20.0	1.0	6.0	125	50
Shredded Wheat	50 g.	177	5.0	1.0	40.0	2	174
Egg whites	100 g.	51	10.9	0.0	0.8	146	139
MCFA Oil	4 Tbsp.	456					
Subtotal		789	35.9	2.0	46.8	273	363
11 A.M.							
Chicken Breast	150 g.	176	35.1	2.9	0.0	75	480
Potato	125 g.	95	2.6	0.1	85.3	3	440
Asparagus	125 g.	33	3.1	0.3	6.3	3	348
Salad	300 g.	69	3.3	0.3	14.4	48	780
MCFA Oil	3.5 Tbsp.	399					
Subtotal		771	44.2	3.5	105.9	128	2,048
1 P.M.							
Halibut	150 g.	150	31.4	1.8	0.0	81	674
Brown Rice	75 g.	270	5.6	1.4	58.2	7	161
Corn	75 g.	72	2.6	0.8	16.6	0	210
Green Beans	75 g.	24	1.4	0.2	5.3	5	182
MCFA Oil	3 Tbsp.	342					
Subtotal		858	41.0	4.1	80.1	93	1,226
3 P.M.							
Haddock	150 g.	119	27.5	0.2	0.0	92	456
Black-eyed Peas	100 g.	131	9.0	0.4	23.6	50	387
Broccoli	150 g.	48	5.4	0.5	8.9	23	423
Salad	300 g.	69	3.3	0.3	14.4	48	780
MCFA Oil	3 Tbsp.	342					
Subtotal		709	45.2	1.3	46.9	212	2,046
Carbohydrate Supplement (during and after workout)							
	2 Scps.	210	8.0	0.0	44.0	128	344
6 P.M.							
Cod	150 g.	117	26.4	0.5	0.0	107	573
Sweet Potato	100 g.	114	1.7	0.4	26.3	10	243
Cauliflower	125 g.	34	3.4	0.3	6.5	16	369
Lima Beans	75 g.	77	4.7	0.1	14.6	97	368
Salad	150 g.	35	1.7	0.2	7.2	24	390
MCFA Oil	3 Tbsp.	342					
Subtotal		718	37.8	1.3	54.6	254	1,942
8 P.M.							
Turkey Breast	125 g.	145	30.8	1.5	0.0	64	400
Broccoli	150 g.	48	5.4	0.5	8.9	23	423
Zucchini	175 g.	30	2.1	0.2	6.3	2	354
Salad	150 g.	35	1.7	0.2	7.2	24	390
MCFA Oil	3.5 Tbsp.	399					
Subtotal		656	39.9	2.3	22.4	112	1,567
Daily Totals		4,711	251.9	14.6	400.6	1,199	9,536

6,000 CALORIES

Time/Food	Amt.	Calories	Protein/g	Fat/g	Carbs/g	Na/mg	K/mg
8 A.M.							
Protein Pwd.	2 Scp.	210	40.0	2.0	12.0	250	100
Oatmeal	50 g.	195	7.1	3.7	34.1	1	176
Egg whites	100 g.	51	10.9	0.0	0.8	146	139
MCFA Oil	5 Tbsp.	570					
Subtotal		1,026	58.0	5.7	46.9	397	415

By following proper nutrition, Bob Cicherillo can train with super intensity, even during pre-contest dieting.
Photo by Jim Amentler.

6,000 CALORIES (Continued)

Time/Food	Amt.	Calories	Protein/g	Fat/g	Carbs/g	Na/mg	K/mg
11 A.M.							
Chicken Breast	150 g.	176	35.1	2.9	0.0	75	480
Potato	150 g.	114	3.2	0.2	102.3	3	528
Asparagus	200 g.	52	5.0	0.4	10.0	4	556
Salad	400 g.	92	4.4	0.4	19.2	64	1,040
MCFA Oil	5 Tbsp.	570					
Subtotal		1,004	47.7	3.8	131.5	146	2,604
1 P.M.							
Halibut	125 g.	125	26.1	1.5	0.0	68	561
Brown Rice	100 g.	360	7.5	1.9	77.6	9	214
Corn	100 g.	96	3.5	1.0	22.1	0	280
Green Beans	125 g.	40	2.4	0.3	8.9	9	304
MCFA Oil	4.5 Tbsp.	513					
Subtotal		1,134	39.5	4.7	108.6	85	1,359
3 P.M.							
Haddock	125 g.	99	22.9	0.1	0.0	76	380
Black-eyed Peas	150 g.	197	13.5	0.6	35.4	75	581
Broccoli	225 g.	72	8.1	0.7	13.3	34	635
Salad	200 g.	46	2.2	0.2	9.6	32	520
MCFA Oil	5 Tbsp.	570					
Subtotal		983	46.7	1.6	58.3	217	2,115
Carbohydrate Supplement (during and after workout)							
	2 Scps.	210	8.0	0.0	44.0	128	344
6 P.M.							
Cod	125 g.	98	22.0	0.4	0.0	89	478
Sweet Potato	150 g.	171	2.6	0.6	39.5	15	365
Cauliflower	175 g.	47	4.7	0.4	9.1	23	516
Lima Beans	100 g.	102	6.2	0.1	19.5	129	490
Salad	200 g.	46	2.2	0.2	9.6	32	520
MCFA Oil	4.5 Tbsp.	513					
Subtotal		977	37.7	1.6	77.7	288	2,368
8 P.M.							
Turkey Breast	200 g.	232	49.2	2.4	0.0	102	640
Broccoli	150 g.	48	5.4	0.5	8.9	23	423
Zucchini	200 g.	34	2.4	0.2	7.2	2	404
MCFA Oil	5 Tbsp.	570					
Subtotal		884	57.0	3.1	16.1	127	1,467
Daily Totals		6,218	294.5	20.4	483.0	1,387	10,672

8,000 CALORIES

Time/Food	Amt.	Calories	Protein/g	Fat/g	Carbs/g	Na/mg	K/mg
8 A.M.							
Protein Pwd.	2 Scps.	210	40.0	2.0	12.0	250	100
Oatmeal	100 g.	390	14.2	7.4	68.2	2	352
Egg whites	100 g.	51	10.9	0.0	0.8	146	139
MCFA Oil	6 Tbsp.	684					
Subtotal		1,335	65.1	9.4	81.0	398	591
11 A.M.							
Chicken Breast	150 g.	176	35.1	2.9	0.0	75	480
Potato	225 g.	171	4.7	0.2	153.5	5	792
Asparagus	225 g.	59	5.6	0.5	11.3	5	626
Salad	200 g.	46	2.2	0.2	9.6	32	520
MCFA Oil	7 Tbsp.	798					
Subtotal		1,249	47.7	3.7	174.3	116	2,418
1 P.M.							
Halibut	125 g.	125	26.1	1.5	0.0	68	561
Brown Rice	100 g.	360	7.5	1.9	77.6	9	214
Corn	100 g.	96	3.5	1.0	22.1	0	280
Green Beans	125 g.	40	2.4	0.3	8.9	9	304
MCFA Oil	6 Tbsp.	684					
Subtotal		1,305	39.5	4.7	108.6	85	1,359

Time/Food	Amt.	Calories	Protein/g	Fat/g	Carbs/g	Na/mg	K/mg
3 P.M.							
Haddock	125 g.	99	22.9	0.1	0.0	76	380
Black-eyed Peas	200 g.	262	18.0	0.8	47.2	100	774
Broccoli	225 g.	72	8.1	0.7	13.3	34	635
Salad	200 g.	46	2.2	0.2	9.6	32	520
MCFA Oil	6 Tbsp.	684					
Subtotal		1,163	51.2	1.8	70.1	242	2,309
Carbohydrate Supplement (during and after workout)							
	4 Scps.	420	16.0	0.0	88.0	256	688
6 P.M.							
Cod	150 g.	117	26.4	0.5	0.0	107	573
Sweet Potato	225 g.	257	3.8	0.9	59.2	23	547
Cauliflower	175 g.	47	4.7	0.4	9.1	23	516
Lima Beans	100 g.	102	6.2	0.1	19.5	129	490
Salad	200 g.	46	2.2	0.2	9.6	32	520
MCFA Oil	5.5 Tbsp.	627					
Subtotal		1,196	43.4	2.0	97.4	313	2,646
8 P.M.							
Turkey Breast	250 g.	290	61.5	3.0	0.0	128	800
Broccoli	225 g.	72	8.1	0.7	13.3	34	635
Zucchini	200 g.	34	2.4	0.2	7.2	2	404
MCFA Oil	6 Tbsp.	684					
Subtotal		1,080	72.0	3.9	20.5	163	1,839
Daily Totals		7,748	334.8	25.5	639.8	1,573	11,849

Getting Lean: Stage 2

Stage 2 lasts approximately four weeks and is designed to further tighten up your physique and promote body fat loss at the rate of one pound a week. In Stage 2, reduce your number of meals from six to five. Eat your last meal three to four hours before going to bed. Decrease your intake of starchy carbohydrates even more at all meals, except your pre-workout meal. Consume larger portions of fibrous carbohydrates.

Continue your accelerated program of aerobics but never run out of energy. If you do, eat a few more starchy carbohydrates. Increase your intake of MCFA oil too. This is a source of calories your body can use for fuel. It has very little tendency to be stored as fat because of its rapid absorption, high thermic effect, conversion to ketones, and ability to be burned in a carbohydrate-loaded cell.

To sum up Stage 2:
Reduce your meals from six to five.
Reduce your intake of starchy carbohydrates.

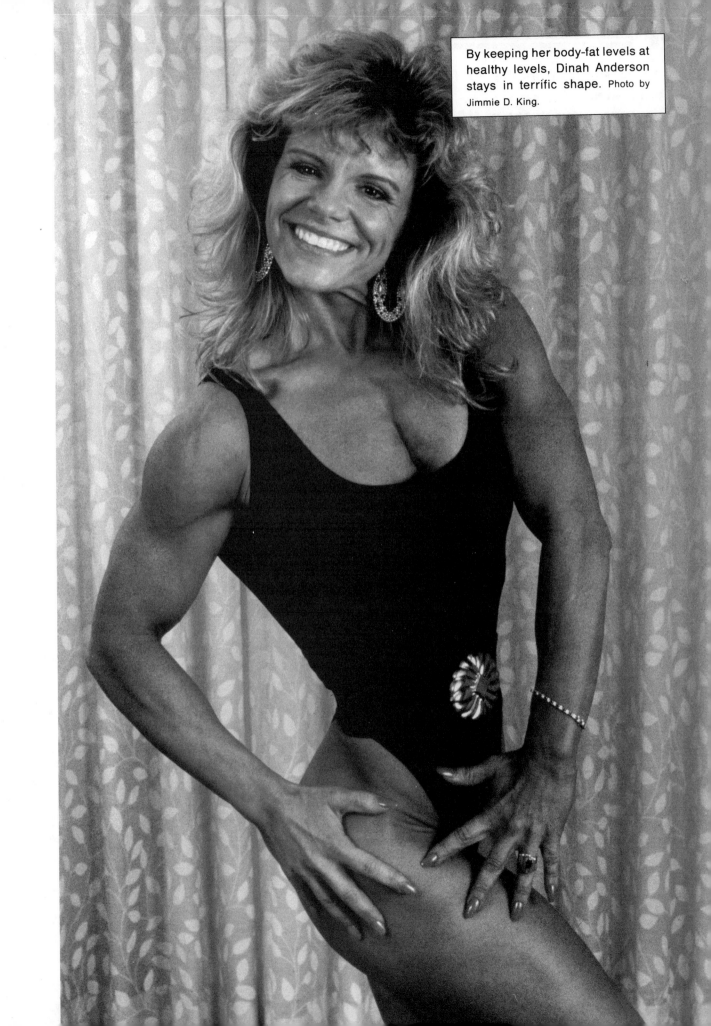

By keeping her body-fat levels at healthy levels, Dinah Anderson stays in terrific shape. Photo by Jimmie D. King.

Increase your intake of fibrous carbohydrates.
Increase your usage of MCFA oil.

Stage 2 Menus

Here are sample menus for Stage 2:

2,000 CALORIES

Time/Food	Amt.	Calories	Protein/g	Fat/g	Carbs/g	Na/mg	K/mg
8 A.M.							
Protein Pwd.	1 Scp.	105	20.0	1.0	6.0	125	50
Oatmeal	25 g.	98	3.6	1.9	17.1	1	88
Egg whites	100 g.	51	10.9	0.0	0.8	146	139
MCFA Oil	0.5 Tbsp.	57					
Subtotal		311	34.5	2.9	23.9	272	277
11 A.M.							
Chicken Breast	150 g.	176	35.1	2.9	0.0	75	480
Broccoli	25 g.	8	0.9	0.1	1.5	4	71
Asparagus	50 g.	13	1.3	0.1	2.5	1	139
Salad	150 g.	35	1.7	0.2	7.2	24	390
MCFA Oil	2 Tbsp.	228					
Subtotal		460	38.9	3.2	11.2	104	1,080
2 P.M.							
Halibut	150 g.	150	31.4	1.8	0.0	81	674
Zucchini	100 g.	17	1.2	0.1	3.6	1	202
Green Beans	25 g.	8	0.5	0.1	1.8	2	61
MCFA Oil	0.5 Tbsp.	57					
Subtotal		232	33.0	2.0	5.4	84	936
5 P.M.							
Haddock	175 g.	138	32.0	0.2	0.0	107	532
Asparagus	25 g.	7	0.6	0.1	1.3	1	70
Broccoli	25 g.	8	0.9	0.1	1.5	4	71
Salad	300 g.	69	3.3	0.3	14.4	48	780
MCFA Oil	2 Tbsp.	228					
Subtotal		450	36.9	0.6	17.1	159	1,452
8 P.M.							
Cod	50 g.	117	26.4	0.5	0.0	107	573
Zucchini	100 g.	17	1.2	0.1	3.6	1	202
Cauliflower	100 g.	27	2.7	0.2	5.2	13	295
Salad	300 g.	69	3.3	0.3	14.4	48	780
MCFA Oil	2 Tbsp.	228					
Subtotal		458	33.6	1.1	23.2	169	1,850
Daily Totals		1,911	176.8	9.6	80.7	787	5,595

2,500 CALORIES

Time/Food	Amt.	Calories	Protein/g	Fat/g	Carbs/g	Na/mg	K/mg
8 A.M.							
Protein Pwd.	1 Scp.	105	20.0	1.0	6.0	125	50
Oatmeal	25 g.	98	3.6	1.9	17.1	1	88
Egg whites	100 g.	51	10.9	0.0	0.8	146	139
MCFA Oil	2 Tbsp.	228					
Subtotal		482	34.5	2.9	23.9	272	277
11 A.M.							
Chicken Breast	150 g.	176	35.1	2.9	0.0	75	480
Cauliflower	50 g.	14	1.4	0.1	2.6	7	148
Asparagus	50 g.	13	1.3	0.1	2.5	1	139
Salad	300 g.	69	3.3	0.3	14.4	48	780
MCFA Oil	2 Tbsp.	228					
Subtotal		499	41.0	3.4	19.5	131	1,547
2 P.M.							
Halibut	150 g.	150	31.4	1.8	0.0	81	674
Zucchini	100 g.	17	1.2	0.1	3.6	1	202
Green Beans	100 g.	32	1.9	0.2	7.1	7	243
MCFA Oil	1 Tbsp.	114					
Subtotal		313	34.5	2.1	10.7	89	1,119
5 P.M.							
Cod	175 g.	137	30.8	0.5	0.0	124	669
Asparagus	50 g.	13	1.3	0.1	2.5	1	139
Cauliflower	50 g.	14	1.4	0.1	2.6	7	148
MCFA Oil	4 Tbsp.	456					
Subtotal		619	33.4	0.7	5.1	132	955
8 P.M.							
Turkey Breast	100 g.	116	24.6	1.2	0.0	51	320
Broccoli	75 g.	24	2.7	0.2	4.4	11	212
Zucchini	100 g.	17	1.2	0.1	3.6	1	202
Salad	300 g.	69	3.3	0.3	14.4	48	780
MCFA Oil	4 Tbsp.	456					
Subtotal		682	31.8	1.8	22.4	111	1,514
Daily Totals		2,595	175.1	10.9	81.6	734	5,411

3,500 CALORIES

Time/Food	Amt.	Calories	Protein/g	Fat/g	Carbs/g	Na/mg	K/mg
8 A.M.							
Protein Pwd.	1 Scp.	105	20.0	1.0	6.0	125	50
Shredded Wheat	50 g.	177	5.0	1.0	40.0	2	174
Egg whites	100 g.	51	10.9	0.0	0.8	146	139
MCFA Oil	4 Tbsp.	456					
Subtotal		789	35.9	2.0	46.8	273	363
11 A.M.							
Chicken Breast	150 g.	176	35.1	2.9	0.0	75	480
Zucchini	175 g.	30	2.1	0.2	6.3	2	354
Asparagus	125 g.	33	3.1	0.3	6.3	3	348
Salad	300 g.	69	3.3	0.3	14.4	48	780
MCFA Oil	4 Tbsp.	456					
Subtotal		763	43.6	3.6	27.0	127	1,961
2 P.M.							
Halibut	150 g.	150	31.4	1.8	0.0	81	674
Broccoli	150 g.	48	5.4	0.5	8.9	23	423
Green Beans	75 g.	24	1.4	0.2	5.3	5	182
MCFA Oil	4 Tbsp.	456					
Subtotal		678	38.2	2.4	14.2	109	1,279
5 P.M.							
Cod	150 g.	117	26.4	0.5	0.0	107	573
Cauliflower	125 g.	34	3.4	0.3	6.5	16	369
Asparagus	125 g.	33	3.1	0.3	6.3	3	348
MCFA Oil	4 Tbsp.	456					
Subtotal		639	32.9	1.0	12.8	125	1,289
8 P.M.							
Turkey Breast	125 g.	145	30.8	1.5	0.0	64	400
Broccoli	150 g.	48	5.4	0.5	8.9	23	423
Zucchini	175 g.	30	2.1	0.2	6.3	2	354
Salad	150 g.	35	1.7	0.2	7.2	24	390
MCFA Oil	4 Tbsp.	456					
Subtotal		713	39.9	2.3	22.4	112	1,567
Daily Totals		3,582	190.5	11.2	123.0	746	6,459

5,000 CALORIES

Time/Food	Amt.	Calories	Protein/g	Fat/g	Carbs/g	Na/mg	K/mg
8 A.M.							
Protein Pwd.	2 Scps.	210	40.0	2.0	12.0	250	100
Oatmeal	50 g.	195	7.1	3.7	34.1	1	176
Egg whites	100 g.	51	10.9	0.0	0.8	146	139
MCFA Oil	5 Tbsp.	570					
Subtotal		1,026	58.0	5.7	46.9	397	415
11 A.M.							
Chicken Breast	150 g.	176	35.1	2.9	0.0	75	480
Cauliflower	175 g.	47	4.7	0.4	9.1	23	516
Asparagus	200 g.	52	5.0	0.4	10.0	4	556
Salad	200 g.	46	2.2	0.2	9.6	32	520
MCFA Oil	6 Tbsp.	684					
Subtotal		1,005	47.0	3.8	28.7	134	2,072
2 P.M.							
Halibut	125 g.	125	26.1	1.5	0.0	68	561
Zucchini	200 g.	34	2.4	0.2	7.2	2	404
Green Beans	125 g.	40	2.4	0.3	8.9	9	304
MCFA Oil	6 Tbsp.	684					
Subtotal		883	30.9	2.0	16.1	78	1,269
5 P.M.							
Cod	125 g.	98	22.0*	0.4	0.0	89	478
Broccoli	150 g.	48	5.4	0.5	8.9	23	423
Cauliflower	175 g.	47	4.7	0.4	9.1	23	516
Salad	200 g.	46	2.2	0.2	9.6	32	520
MCFA Oil	6 Tbsp.	684					
Subtotal		923	34.3	1.4	27.6	166	1,937
8 P.M.							
Turkey Breast	200 g.	232	49.2	2.4	0.0	102	640
Broccoli	150 g.	48	5.4	0.5	8.9	23	423
Zucchini	200 g.	34	2.4	0.2	7.2	2	404
MCFA Oil	6 Tbsp.	684					
Subtotal		998	57.0	3.1	16.1	127	1,467
Daily Totals		4,835	227.3	15.9	135.3	902	7,160

6,000 CALORIES

Time/Food	Amt.	Calories	Protein/g	Fat/g	Carbs/g	Na/mg	K/mg
8 A.M.							
Protein Pwd.	2 Scps.	210	40.0	2.0	12.0	250	100
Oatmeal	50 g.	195	7.1	3.7	34.1	1	176
Egg whites	100 g.	51	10.9	0.0	0.8	146	139
MCFA Oil	7 Tbsp.	798					
Subtotal		1,254	58.0	5.7	46.9	397	415
11 A.M.							
Chicken Breast	150 g.	176	35.1	2.9	0.0	75	480
Cauliflower	175 g.	47	4.7	0.4	9.1	23	516
Asparagus	225 g.	59	5.6	0.5	11.3	5	626
Salad	200 g.	46	2.2	0.2	9.6	32	520
MCFA Oil	7 Tbsp.	798					
Subtotal		1,125	47.7	3.9	30.0	134	2,142
2 P.M.							
Halibut	125 g.	125	26.1	1.5	0.0	68	561
Zucchini	200 g.	34	2.4	0.2	7.2	2	404
Green Beans	125 g.	40	2.4	0.3	8.9	9	304
MCFA Oil	7 Tbsp.	798					
Subtotal		997	30.9	2.0	16.1	78	1,269
5 P.M.							
Cod	150 g.	117	26.4	0.5	0.0	107	573
Asparagus	225 g.	59	5.6	0.5	11.3	5	626
Cauliflower	175 g.	47	4.7	0.4	9.1	23	516
Salad	200 g.	46	2.2	0.2	9.6	32	520
MCFA Oil	8 Tbsp.	912					
Subtotal		1,181	39.0	1.5	30.0	166	2,235
8 P.M.							
Turkey Breast	250 g.	290	61.5	3.0	0.0	128	800
Broccoli	225 g.	72	8.1	0.7	13.3	34	635
Zucchini	200 g.	34	2.4	0.2	7.2	2	404
MCFA Oil	8 Tbsp.	912					
Subtotal		1,308	72.0	3.9	20.5	163	1,839
Daily Totals		5,865	247.5	16.8	143.4	939	7,899

Getting Lean: Stage 3 (For Competitive Bodybuilders)

Stage 3 lasts two weeks. Designed for competitive bodybuilders who want to achieve peak contest shape, Stage 3 is the time to polish your physique, tighten it up, and rid yourself of any water that lies underneath the skin.

In Stage 3, follow the same meal plan you used in Stage 2—with one exception. Further reduce your intake of starchy carbohydrates, so that you lose your pump about two-thirds to three-fourths of the way through your workout. If you're already experiencing this, there is no need to make any adjustments in your carbohydrate intake.

The week before your contest, practice "decarbing" and "carbing up." Decarbing is the process of lowering your carbohydrate intake for several days early in the week. This results in the depletion of glycogen stores, thus preparing your body to hold glycogen and fluid in the muscles rather than under the skin.

To decarb, start lowering your intake of starchy carbohydrates on the Sunday before your contest and continue through Wednesday. Women with slower metabolisms may have to go as low as 50 grams of carbohydrates a day; with faster metabolisms, 100 to 200 grams a day. Men with slower metabolisms will have to lower their carbohydrates to 100 to 200 grams a day; with faster metabolisms, to 200 to 400 grams a day. During decarbing, use MCFA oil to supply energy and to assist in fat-burning.

Decarbing is followed by a period of "carbing up" in which you reintroduce starchy carbohydrates such as potatoes and brown rice into your diet. Carbing up rebuilds glycogen stores in your muscles so that you look full, hard, and well-defined on contest day. Increasing your carbohydrate intake, while watching your fluid intake, draws the interstitial water out from under your skin, and your body will tighten up considerably as a result.

On Thursday before a Saturday contest, start reintroducing carbs into your meals at the rate of 50 to 200 grams a day for women and 100 to 400 grams a day for men. The rate at which you add carbs back in depends on your metabolism and energy levels. The additional carbs should be divided equally among your five, six, or more meals.

Stage 3: Overcoming Water Retention

Regulating water intake is a critical factor for competitive bodybuilders in Stage 3. Regardless of how well you dieted or how hard you trained, water retention can wash away all your hopes for peak condition. Holding too much water, you look puffy, smooth, and flat.

Water retention is caused by a number of factors, including cytoxic (allergic) reactions to certain foods, overconsumption of carbohydrates and water, or an imbalance of sodium (taking in too much or too little). Desperate to avoid water retention, some bodybuilders take the easy way out: They use diuretics on contest day. These flush precious electrolytes from your system, leading to muscle cramping, dizziness, and other ill effects. Even electrolyte-sparing diuretics are dangerous when abused this way. They rob your body of sodium—a depletion that also causes cramping and other side effects.

Still other bodybuilders totally restrict water. In this dehydrated state, the body hoards water even more, and the physique becomes bloated as a result.

You can control water retention—and do it in a safe way—so that you enter your contest looking hard and ripped. Here are some proven methods to help you prevent water retention:

Monitor water intake. On the last day before your contest, drink six ounces of water with each of your meals. In the body, water combines with glucose, derived from carbohydrates, to manufacture glycogen. Stored in the muscles, glycogen makes muscles look hard and full. Without adequate intake of water or carbs, you'll look flat, rather than hard, tight, and vascular. This amount of water will keep you slightly water-deficient—a condition which also draws the interstitial water out from under the skin for a harder, tighter look.

Monitor your sodium and potassium intake. Many competitors mistakenly believe that they must completely eliminate sodium from their diet. Actually, you need some sodium—between 500 mg. and one gram a day—to look hard and full. This amount should be naturally present in the foods you eat while carbing up.

The trick is to keep your sodium/potassium ratio in balance. By carbing up on natural carbohydrates, you take in high amounts of potassium. If there's too little sodium in your system, your body accelerates its production of aldosterone, a hormone that regulates the vital sodium/potassium balance. Inadequate concentrations of sodium can actually make you look smooth.

Ms. Olympia Lenda Murray diets to win. Photo by J. M. Manion.

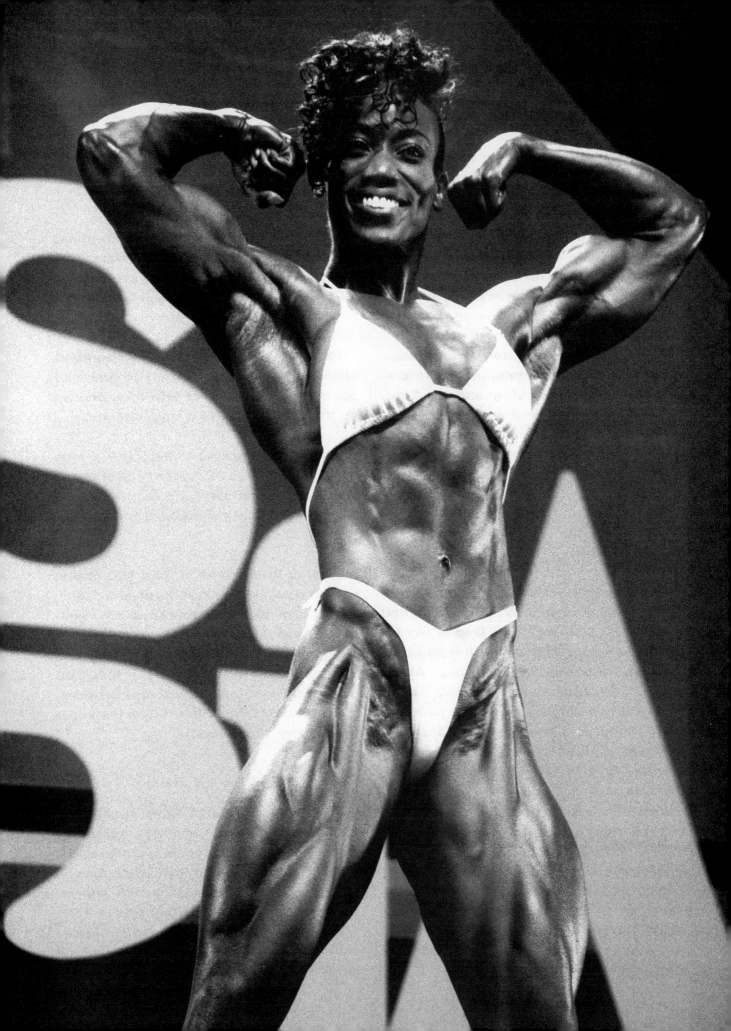

Avoid any foods which cause cytoxic reactions. These include wheat and dairy products—foods which can result in puffiness.

Be careful about the type of water you drink prior to your contest. Some city water supplies are high in electrolytes such as sodium and calcium, which can both result in puffiness when taken in excess. If you're drinking water from a water supply other than what you're used to, take your own water with you to the contest—provided that water has not made you retain water in the past.

If your drinking water does cause water-retention problems, switch to distilled water for drinking and cooking. When drinking distilled water, however, be sure to take mineral-electrolyte supplements, because distilled water contains no minerals.

A DIET TO WIN

I have worked with many competitors, helping them plan their off-season and pre-contest training diets. One of my favorites is Lenda Murray, who now holds two consecutive Ms. Olympia titles. At her first Ms. Olympia contest in 1990, Lenda so overwhelmed the audience with her cuts, shape, and posing routine that she received a standing ovation and an encore—a first in the history of the Ms. Olympia.

Weighing a lean off-season weight of 157 pounds, Lenda started her diet 12 weeks before the contest, giving her ample time to reach her contest weight of 145 pounds. As reported in the July 1991 issue of *MuscleMag International* by writer Carol Ann Weber, Lenda's diet illustrates exactly how the 12-week, three-stage system works:

Stage 1 (Used for 6 weeks)

Meal 1: 100 grams of oatmeal, 4 egg whites, 1 cup of coffee, and supplements (multivitamin supplement, multimineral supplement, lipotropics, nutritional GH releasers, and amino acids).

Meal 2: 200 grams of white-meat chicken, 120 grams of baked potato, 100 grams of a green vegetable, 2½ tbsp. of MCFA oil poured on the vegetables, and supplements (same as above).

Meal 3: 200 grams of white-meat chicken, 100 grams of rice, 100 grams of asparagus, 2½ tbsp. of MCFA oil poured on the vegetables, and supplements.

Meal 4: 200 grams of fish, 150 grams of baked potato, 100 grams each of green beans and cauliflower, 2½ tbsp. of MCFA oil poured on the vegetables, and supplements.

Meal 5: 200 grams of fish, 150 grams of baked potato, 100 grams of asparagus, 2½ tbsp. of MCFA oil poured on the vegetables, and supplements.

Meal 6: 250 to 300 grams of fish, 100 grams each of asparagus and broccoli, 2½ tbsp. of MCFA oil poured on the vegetables, and supplements.

Stage 2 (Used for 4 Weeks)

At this stage, Lenda modified her Stage 1 diet by excluding rice and baked potatoes (her starchy carbohydrates) from meals. Her only source of starchy carbohydrates was her meal-1 oatmeal, which she increased slightly from 100 grams to 150–200 grams. Additionally, Lenda eliminated her sixth meal and increased her MCFA oil to 3 ½ tablespoons per meal.

Stage 3 (Used for 2 Weeks)

Lenda's daily meal plan was the same one used in Stage 2. The week before the show, she decarbed by eliminating her meal-1 oatmeal on Sunday, Monday, Tuesday, and Wednesday. She also began drinking more water. On Wednesday, she stopped using MCFA oil.

Lenda began carbing up on Thursday, Friday, and Saturday (the day of the show) by adding in about 50 grams of a starchy carbohydrate (usually sweet potatoes) at each of her five meals. On Saturday, she cut her starchy carbs back to 100 grams and drank a minimal amount of water.

Reach Your Peak

On the day of your own contest, scrutinize your physique. If your muscles are hard but your skin is loose, drink slightly less water. If your muscles are soft and lack vascularity, increase your carbohydrates and slightly more water. On the other hand, if you look hard, ripped, and vascular, do not change a thing. You have achieved contest-winning appearance.

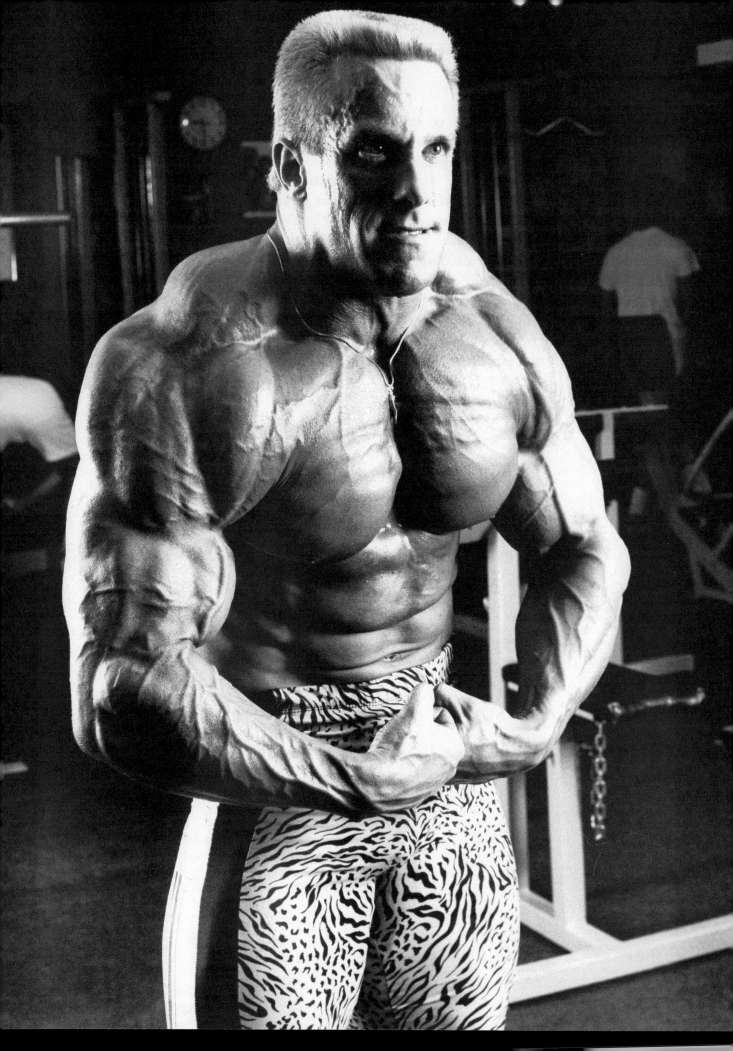

EIGHT
THE BIOMECHANICS OF BUILDING MASS

The name of the game in bodybuilding is lean mass. You build it by combining scientific principles of nutrition and supplementation with strict training designed to push every muscle fiber to its absolute limit.

Many bodybuilders believe that overloading the muscle with increasingly heavier weight is the chief way to build greater mass. Without question, progressive, heavy weight training does pack on mass, as long you're eating properly and taking the right nutritional supplements. But there's another issue involved—one that often goes neglected, even among the most experienced bodybuilders. That issue is proper biomechanics (strict form), and it can make the critical difference between gains that are just so-so and those that are phenomenal.

My method of training involves five distinct and essential elements of proper biomechanics, each designed to maximize the efficiency of the movement and elicit a greater adaptive response from the muscle.

Dean Caputo is one of the most muscular competitors around. Photo by J. M. Manion.

PROPERLY ALIGN YOUR MUSCLES PRIOR TO THE EXERCISE.

This means correct positioning of the muscle or muscle groups to be worked—before you even begin the exercise.

A case in point is the bench press. Most bodybuilders use the strength of their deltoids to push through the exercise. The ultimate result is a well-developed set of delts but flat upper pectorals. To properly work the pectoral region, you must press your shoulders down and back into the bench, while thrusting your chest forward. This subtle adjustment in positioning puts the mechanical advantage on the pectoral muscles, thus properly stressing the muscles. Instructions on how to properly align muscles are given for each exercise described in this book.

USE SLOW, STRICT REPETITIONS IN BOTH THE LIFTING AND LOWERING PHASE OF THE EXERCISE.

When you move too fast through an exercise, inertia—and very little of your own muscle power—is doing the work. So you're not really getting much from the exercise. Plus, fast lifting can be very stressful on your connective tissue. Each repetition should be performed in a slow, controlled fashion throughout the range of motion.

BRING YOUR ANTAGONISTIC MUSCLES INTO PLAY.

Muscles assume different roles, depending on the motion of the exercise. The muscle that produces the primary action is termed the "agonist." An example would be the biceps when it flexes upward in a curl exercise. Where there is an agonist, there is also an "antagonist." This is the muscle which opposes the action of the agonist and must relax as the agonist contracts. Using the curl as an example again, the triceps of the upper arm would be the antagonist in this exercise.

You can make any exercise more effective by actively pulling with the antagonistic muscle group during the lowering or negative portion of the exercise. This technique stimulates more muscle fibers for greater growth.

In addition, keep the working muscles in a constant state of tension throughout the range of motion. This action is another way to provide maximum muscle fiber stimulation.

LOCK OUT ON ALL EXERCISES.

Many bodybuilders like to incorporate partial repetitions and limited range lifts into their routines. In these techniques, the muscle is not worked in a complete range of motion from contraction to extension. As a result, much of the muscle goes unworked.

To get the most from every repetition, lock out each time. This means fully straightening the joint at the top of the movement in the contracted position—but without resting there. Locking out in this manner activates more muscle fibers and allows you to work a muscle through its full range of motion. By locking out, you also work your synergistic muscles (those muscles which assist or stabilize the agonist).

PUT MENTAL EFFORT INTO EVERY REP.

To accomplish all of the above and then some, you must exert tremendous mental effort. The degree to which you can push yourself physically depends not only on your state of nutrition but also on your "mental acuity" or power of mental concentration. The more concentrated your effort, the closer you can get to achieving your goals.

THE 42 BEST EXERCISES FOR MASS AND MUSCULARITY

There are literally hundreds of bodybuilding exercises. In this section, I cover those which I consider the most effective for building mass and muscularity—and the ones which require clarification on the finer points of exercise form. Also included are several exercises which may be new to you.

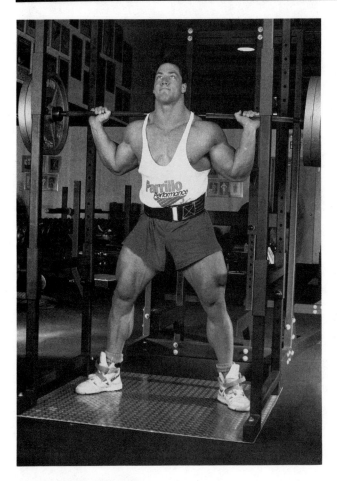 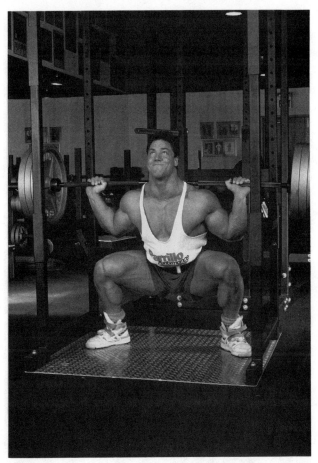

LEG EXERCISES

Squat

Muscles Worked: **Considered one of the best mass-building exercises, the squat directly stresses the quadriceps, a group of four muscles in the frontal thigh; gluteal muscles, a group of three muscles in the hip region (the gluteus maximus, gluteus medius, and gluteus minimus, also known as the "glutes"); and the adductors, the muscles of the inner thigh. Secondary emphasis is placed on the hamstrings, a group of three muscles at the back of the thigh, and the lower back.**

Start: **Squats can be performed in two ways, depending on which area of your thighs you want to work. To build an impressive sweep on your outer thighs, for example, take a wider stance with your toes angled out.**

Action: **Descend slowly to a deep position—past the point at which your thighs are parallel to the floor. Then press up from your heels and drive your hips forward and your knees out. When descending, always sit back. Upon arising, force your knees out and come up under the weight. Keep your legs tight and use your hamstring muscles to pull yourself to the start position. On any squat movement, to keep from straining your lower back, you must push your hips forward and straighten your back as soon as you begin your ascent from the bottom of the movement. The moment your rear end goes up and back, stress is placed on your lower back.**

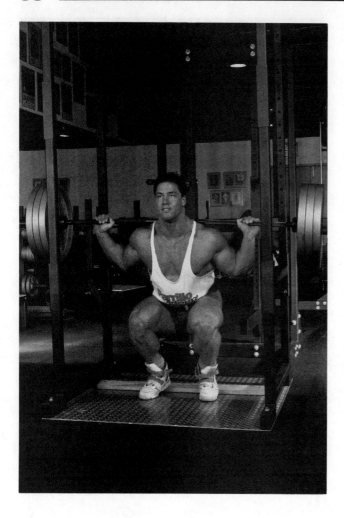

Variation: To emphasize frontal thigh development, stand with your toes pointed forward. Descend slowly, keeping your knees forward. Press up, using the balls of your feet.

Performance points: No matter what area you work, outer sweep or frontal thigh, you must stay tight and practice slow, strict form throughout the exercise. Many bodybuilders make the mistake of relaxing at the bottom of the movement and then bouncing off the bottom of their calves. Such an action can injure the ligaments in your knees.
If you're training for bodybuilding competition, eliminate heavy squatting one to two weeks before the contest. This is so your legs will reduce slightly in size, giving room under the fascia (the tissue surrounding the muscle) for separations and actually making your legs look bigger.

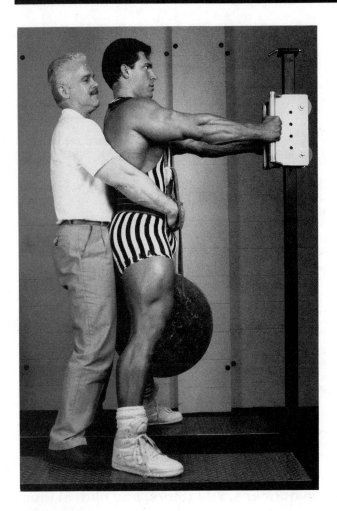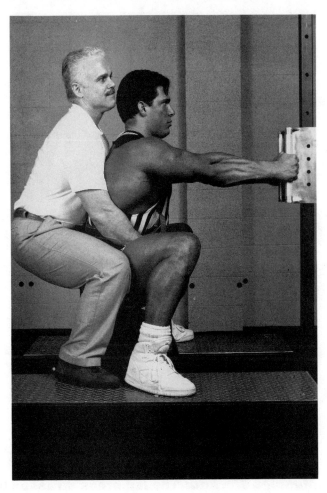

Belt Squat

Muscles Worked: In the belt squat, the entire training load is concentrated on the quadriceps, gluteal muscles, adductors, and hamstrings.

Start: The belt squat requires a special machine, and several types exist. Strap the weight apparatus to your body according to the machine's design. A spotter should stand behind you to smoothly guide you through the movement. Additionally, the spotter helps you center your weight and keeps your momentum going for maximum intensity. Take an upright position and angle your toes outward.

Action: In a steady controlled motion, descend to a deep position, well below parallel. Keep your knees straight out over your toes. Drive your hips forward, pushing your knees out. As you ascend, continue pushing your hips forward. Squeeze your gluteal muscles and complete the movement by locking your knees. Throughout the exercise, always look upward.

Performance Points: The belt squat is one of the safest ways to squat, particularly for athletes recovering from back or knee injuries. The upright position eliminates stress on the lower back and spine and reduces pressure on the knees. You can still train your legs but without placing undue stress on the injured areas.

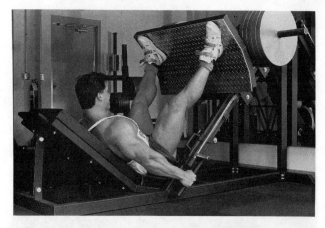
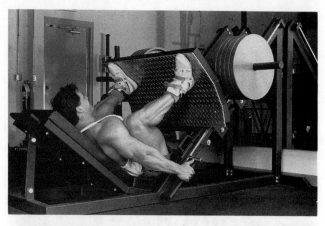
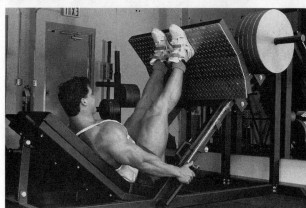
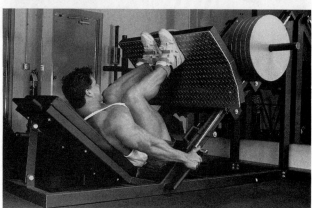

Incline Leg Press

Muscles Worked: The leg press stresses the quadriceps, adductors, and gluteal muscles. With the incline leg press, you can work various angles of your quadriceps by altering the position of your feet on the platform, by changing the width of your stance on the platform, and by changing the point from which you push. If you place your feet high on the platform with a wide stance and push with your heels, the exercise emphasizes your gluteal muscles, hamstrings, and outer sweep of the thighs. Emphasis shifts to your frontal quads when you take a narrow stance, and you push with the balls of your feet.

Start: Place your feet on the platform according to the area you want to stress. Release the stops and bring your knees slowly toward your chest.

Action: Press back up, locking out hard at the top. Come out of the locked position in one smooth, continuous motion. Keep constant tension on your leg muscles as you push through the exercise. Keep your legs tight and always use the strength of your hamstring muscles to return to the start position.

Performance Points: When training bodybuilders on the leg press, I ask them where they want to "burn" their legs. Give me a six-inch region anywhere on their legs, and I can instruct them on how to isolate that specific area. I place a 2 × 4 board against the leg-press platform and under the bodybuilder's heels. Then I have the bodybuilder push with the heels. This isolates the outer thighs. Next, I remove the board and instruct the bodybuilder to push with the balls of the feet. This shifts the stress to the frontal quads. Once you try these techniques yourself, you'll find that you can make your legs grow in any area you want.

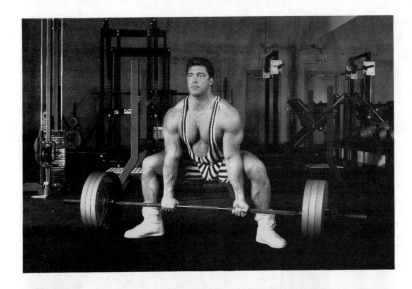

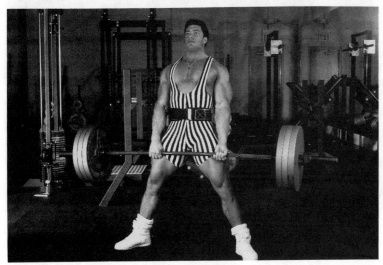

Deadlift

Muscles Worked: **This is an excellent movement for the quadriceps, gluteal muscles, and hamstrings. Secondary stress is placed on the abdominals and the lower back.**

Start: **Take a medium-wide stance. Undergrip the bar in one hand and overgrip it in the other. As you begin to lift the bar, make sure your shoulders move up first. Keep your back slightly arched.**

Action: **Ascend slowly, driving your hips forward. As always, keep your muscles tight throughout the range of motion. Return to start. The same techniques apply to the sumo-style deadlifts, in which a very wide stance is used.**

Performance Points: **Many bodybuilders avoid deadlifts because the exercise can thicken the waist. But often, you need to build your physique to a point beyond where you want to be. Then you can use isolation exercises to sculpt away the thickness, while still holding your size. So for gaining initial size and thickness, deadlifts are an excellent exercise.**

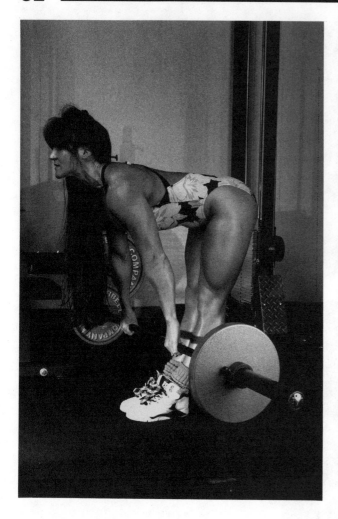
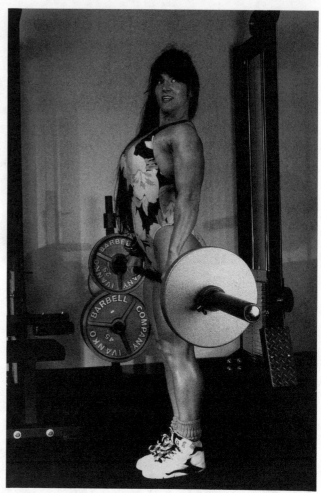

Straight-leg Deadlift

Muscles Worked: My method of performing straight-leg deadlifts is designed to totally isolate the gluteal muscles and hamstrings.

Start: To begin the exercise, bend forward and arch your back. This motion isolates your hamstrings. Stretch your hamstrings at the bottom as you pick up the weight. Keeping your legs straight or slightly bent, slowly lift the bar.

Action: At the top of the movement, tighten your glutes, drive your hips forward, and lock your knees. Then slowly return to the start position, pushing your abdominals toward the floor. Pivot at the hip joint and not with your lower back. Keep everything tight in the process.

Performance Points: Most of the time, you see bodybuilders doing straight-leg deadlifts from a box. You have to be very flexible to do this exercise correctly from a box. A better way to do straight-leg deadlifts is without a box. As long as you pivot at the hip joint and keep your back arched, you should not need to stand on anything. Performed in this manner, straight-leg deadlifts totally isolate the hamstrings and glutes. In fact, there are few other lower body exercises that work these muscles as hard as this one does.

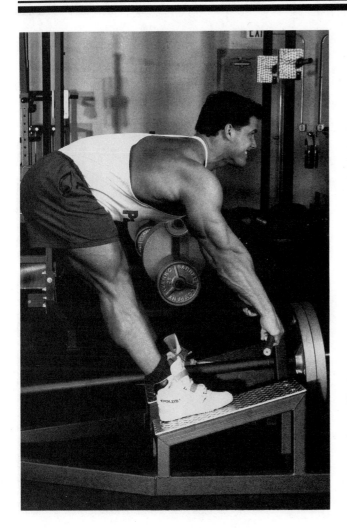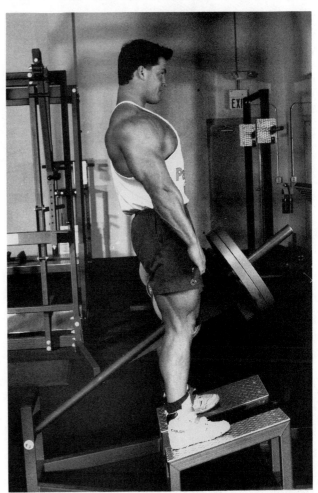

T-Bar Hamstring Lift

Muscles Worked: An alternative to the straight-leg deadlift, this exercise isolates the gluteal muscles and hamstrings and is also an excellent way to stretch these muscles.

Start: This exercise is a combination of T-bar rowing and the straight-leg deadlift. Grip the bar and arch your back. Fully stretch your hamstrings as you begin the exercise.

Action: Pull the bar upward. Pivot at your hip joint, keeping your arms straight. Do not row. At the top of the movement, squeeze your gluteal muscles and hamstrings. Drive your hips forward and lean back slightly for a full contraction. Lower to the start position, keeping constant tension on the working muscles and stretching hard.

Performance Points: By combining the action of the straight-leg deadlift with T-bar rowing, you have another excellent exercise for isolating the glutes. The key is to tighten those muscles at the top.

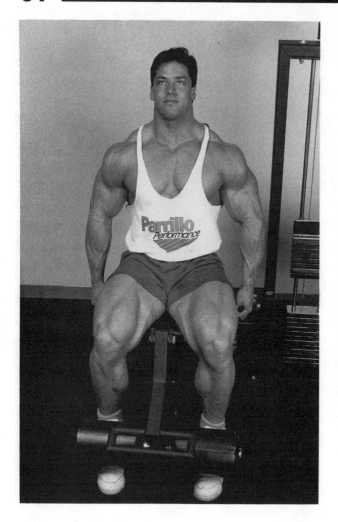 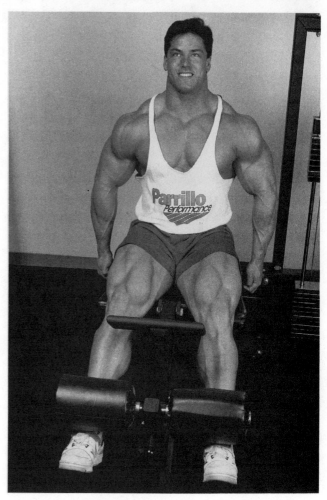

Leg Extensions

Muscles Worked: **This exercise is effective for shaping and defining the frontal quads, particularly the teardrop muscle (the vastus medialis).**

Start: **Hook your insteps under the machine's padded roller. Using strict form, bring your legs upward in an arc.**

Action: **The teardrop muscle is worked the hardest in the last few degrees of the arc, so, at the top of the movement, lock out and squeeze tightly. Make the entire motion smooth and continuous without pausing. Never swing the weight upward. Keep the working muscles tight. Lower slowly to the start position, pulling with your hamstring muscles.**

Performance Points: **Leg extensions are also excellent for strengthening bad knees—as long as you squeeze very hard at the top.**

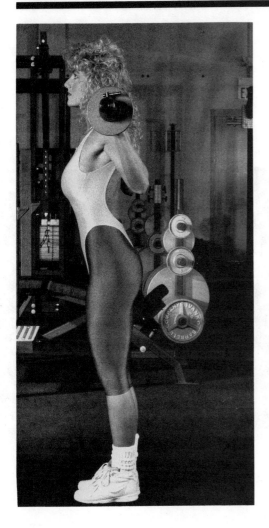

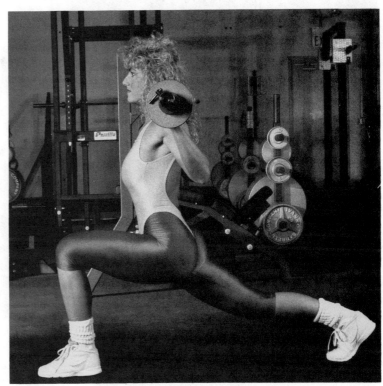

Lunges

Muscles Worked: **The lunge stresses the quadriceps and gluteal muscles, with secondary stress on the hamstrings.**

Start: **Use a light weight, either a barbell or dumbbells. Position the barbell behind your neck and across your shoulders. If you use dumbbells, hold them at your side. Stand with both feet together.**

Action: **Step forward into the lunge, keeping your back leg as straight as possible. Drive your hips forward. Stay tight. Return to the start position and repeat with the other leg.**

Performance Points: **In addition to working the leg muscles, lunges are an excellent exercise because they stretch the entire leg.**

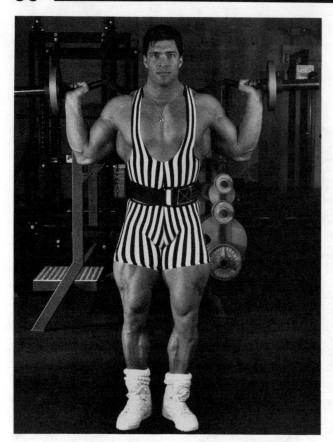

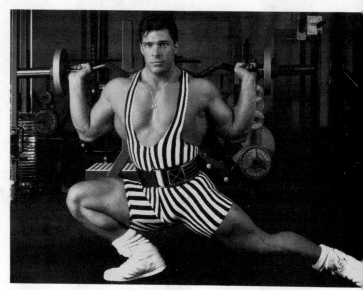

Side Lunges

Muscles Worked: The side lunge works the muscles of the inner thigh, with secondary stress on the quadriceps.

Start: Position the barbell across your shoulders and stand with both feet together.

Action: Step sideways into the lunge, keeping your outstretched leg as straight as you can. Stay tight throughout the movement. Return to the start position and repeat with the other leg.

Performance Points: Like the conventional lunge, the side lunge is a good way to stretch the leg.

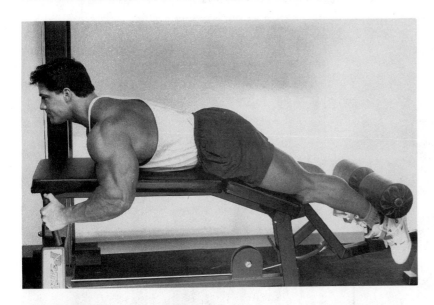

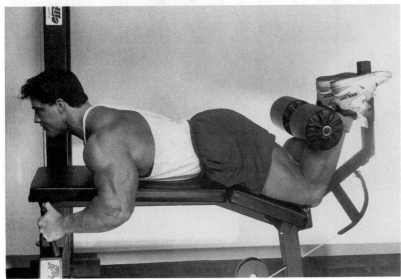

Leg Curls

Muscles Worked: The leg curl isolates the hamstrings and secondarily works the gastrocnemius (the two-headed muscle of the calf).

Start: Lie facedown on the pad and hook your ankles under the padded roller. Press your hips into the pad.

Action: Flex at the knees and curl your legs up toward your hips. Bring the weight all the way to your glutes. Keep your hips pressed into the pad, without raising them up, especially at the top of the movement. Be sure to do this exercise strictly, without jerking the weight. Pull the weight back down, using the strength of your quads. Stay tight.

Performance Points: This exercise can also be performed on a standing leg curl machine in which you work one leg at a time.

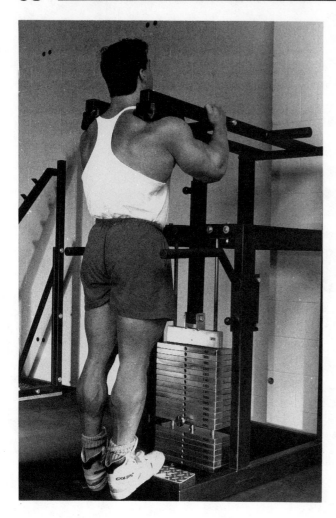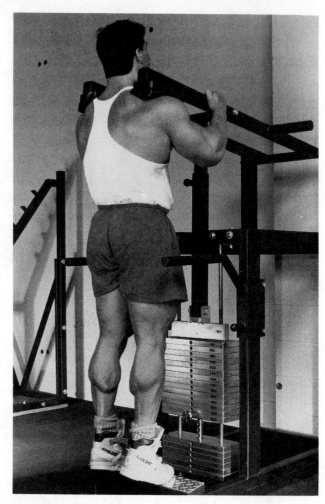

CALF EXERCISES

Standing Calf Raise

Muscles Worked: **The standing calf raise is the best exercise for developing the gastrocnemius.**

Start: **Position your shoulders comfortably under the pads.**

Action: **Raise and lower your heels, striving to get a deep stretch during the movement.**

Performance Points: **By twisting your heels inward at the top of the movement, you'll work the inner head of the gastrocnemius. Twist your heels out at the top, and you'll work the outer head. Lock your knees hard at the top of the movement too. This stresses the gastrocnemius even more.**

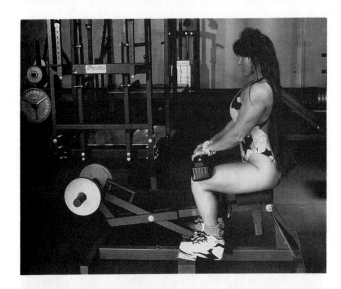

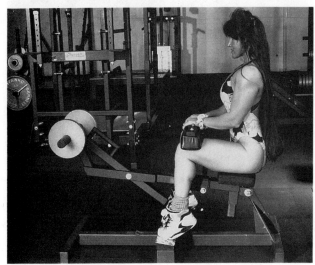

Seated Calf Raise

Muscles Worked: The seated calf raise is the most effective exercise for working the soleus, a supporting muscle located underneath the gastrocnemius.

Start: Typically, you sit in the seated calf machine so that your legs are bent at a 90-degree angle. This position emphasizes the gastrocnemius, however. By breaking the 90-degree angle so that your lower legs are more directly underneath you, you isolate the soleus. As you begin the exercise, make sure the pad fits evenly across your knees to distribute the load properly.

Action: Lift your feet up as high as possible and then lower deeply.

Performance Points: The soleus is a difficult muscle to fatigue because it is comprised primarily of slow-twitch muscle fibers, which are used in endurance activities. So it's a good idea to perform high-rep sets. Between 50 and 100 reps per set are best.

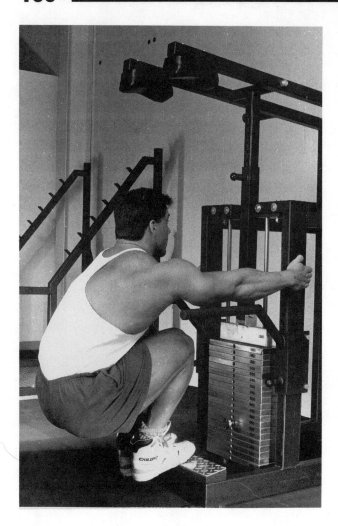 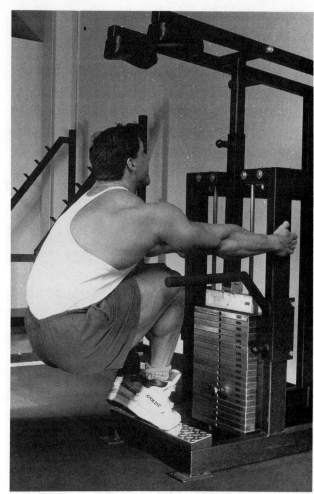

Calf Squats

Muscles Worked: **This exercise is the only way you can totally contract your gastroc-nemius and soleus at the same time.**

Start: **To begin, position the balls of your feet on a block of wood or any elevated platform. For support, grasp a piece of equipment. Squat down, keeping your heels right under your glutes. Press your feet and knees together.**

Action: **Come up as high as you can on the balls of your feet. At the top, press your glutes to your heels. Then lower your feet as deeply as you can, getting a good stretch. Keep everything tight as you return to start.**

Performance Points: **Perform calf squats between sets of standing or seated calf raises for an intense burn in your calf muscles.**

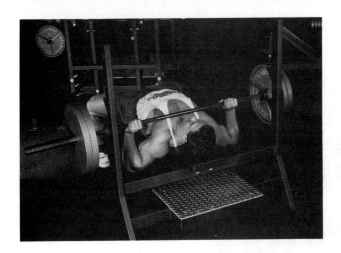 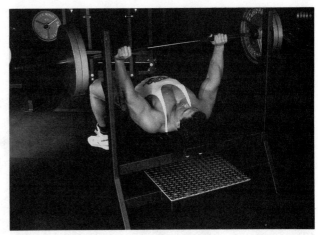

CHEST EXERCISES

Bench Press

Muscles Worked: The bench press builds the pectoralis major and pectoralis minor of the chest, a muscle group also called the pecs. Secondary stress is placed on the triceps, the three-headed muscle of the rear upper arm, and the latissimus dorsi (the lats), the major muscle of the back.

Start: The most important point about bench pressing is to set up your pectoral girdle correctly so that you place the biomechanical advantage squarely on your pecs. Lie back on the bench, take a tight grip, and—this is important—press your shoulders down toward your waist and back into the bench. Then thrust your chest forward and begin the exercise.

Action: At the top of the movement, lock your elbows out. Push your sternum up and squeeze your shoulders down with your lower lats and pec minors. Keep these muscle groups tight throughout the exercise. If you use this form throughout each rep, I guarantee every fiber in your whole chest will burn! Plus, you might discover just how weak your pecs are. Be sure to follow every heavy bench-press set with a special exercise called the Parrillo Dips, which is explained below.

Variation: Another way to perform the bench press is the bench-to-the-neck version, which is excellent for upper-pec development. Take a medium grip on the bar. As with the bench press, it's important to align your pectoral girdle properly to place the biomechanical advantage on your upper pecs. Press your shoulders down toward your waist. Push your sternum up. As you lower the bar, pinch your chin to your chest. Bring the bar down to this pinch point. Then press back up to the starting position, staying tight throughout the entire range of motion.

Performance Points: If you follow my technique for bench pressing, you won't be a "delt bencher." That is what happens when you rely too much on the strength in your front deltoids to push through the exercise. Delt benchers drop their chest at the top of the exercise and then push up with their shoulders. The result? Great front delts but flat, underdeveloped upper pecs.

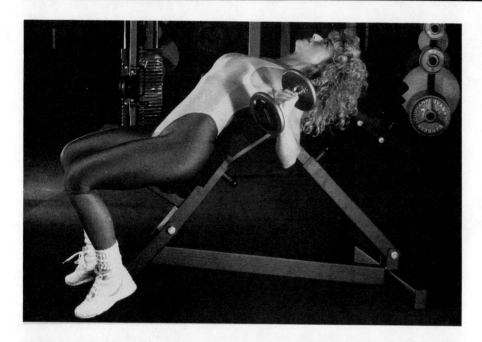

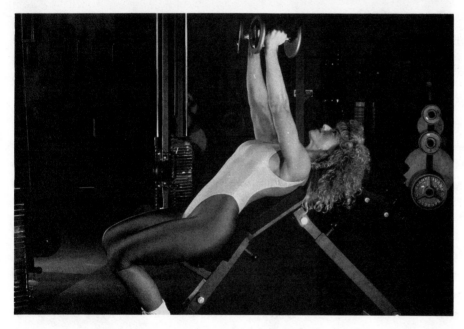

Incline Dumbbell Press

Muscles Worked: **This is an excellent movement for the upper pecs. But if you do it incorrectly, the only muscles you work are your front delts.**

Start: **Lie back on an incline bench. Press your shoulders back into the bench.**

Action: **Press the dumbbells up to an overhead position. At the top of the movement, keep your sternum up and your shoulders down. Push your sternum out as far as possible. Pull the weight slowly to the bottom position, getting a good stretch across your pecs.**

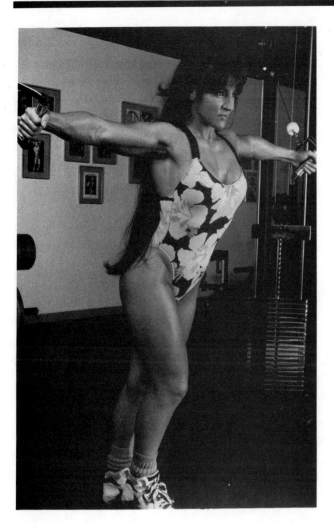 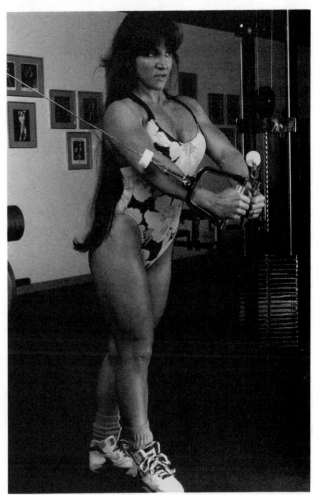

Cable Crossovers

Muscles Worked: **This is an excellent isolation exercise for the pectoralis major and pectoralis minor.**

Start: **Grasp a pulley in each hand, lean forward slightly, and push your chest out.**

Action: **Pull the handles downward in an arc. At the bottom of the movement, push your sternum out. Then hold and squeeze your pecs tightly. Return to the start position and repeat.**

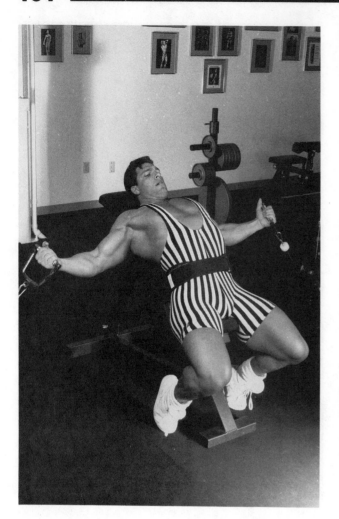 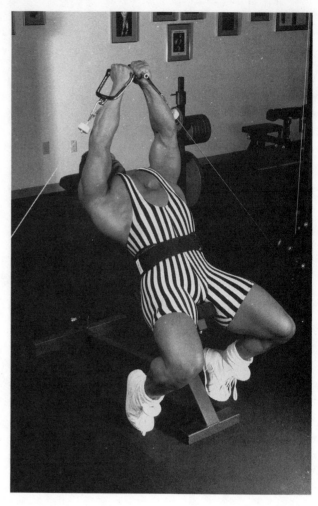

Incline Cable Crossovers

Muscles Worked: **By performing cable crossovers on an incline, you stress your upper pecs.**

Start: **Adjust the pulleys so that they are in the low position. Place an incline bench midway between the pulleys. Take a pulley in each hand and lie on the bench. Keep your shoulders pressed into the bench throughout the movement.**

Action: **Pull the handles upward in an arc. To get full isolation of the pecs, bring your elbows together at the top of the movement. Then push your sternum out at the top. The same technique should be used when performing cable crossovers.**

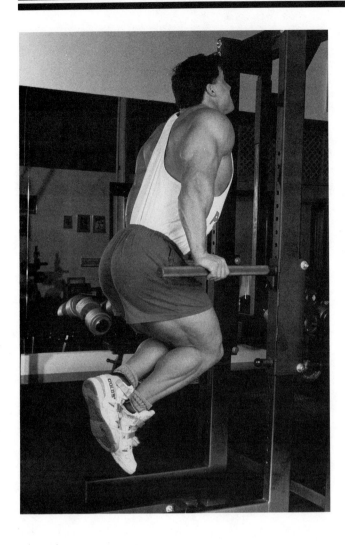

Parrillo Dips

Muscles Worked: This is a special exercise I developed for building the pectoralis minor and lower lats. These muscles support the entire pectoral girdle. By building this support structure, you can keep your pectoral girdle properly aligned when performing heavy chest exercises—a positioning which leads to fuller pectoral development.

Start: Using your arms to support your body, suspend yourself between the dip bars.

Action: Lower your body as far as possible, but without bending your arms. Press back up, pushing your chest out. Squeeze your pecs hard at the top. Pull your knees up to place more emphasis on the chest. Do not bounce.

Performance Points: This exercise should be performed between heavy sets of pectoral exercises.

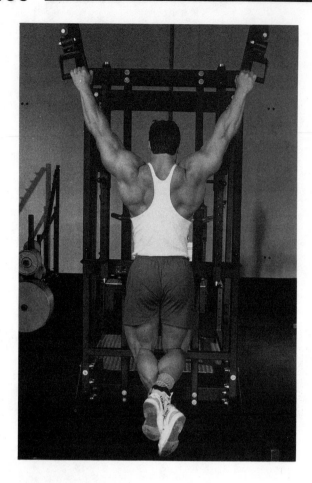 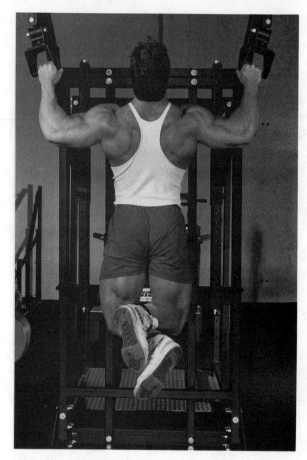

BACK EXERCISES

Pull-ups

Muscles Worked: Performed with the proper biomechanics, this exercise is designed to build the lower lats. However, I see a whole new crop of bodybuilders today with no lower lats—for two reasons. First, they have relied too heavily on machines early in their training. And second, if they include pull-ups in their routines, they usually perform the exercise with too much of an arch in their backs. This common error places stress on the rhomboids and upper lats rather than on the lower lats.

Start: Take an overhand grip on the bar or handles. Keep your knees bent and held out in front of your torso. This position prevents your back from arching and helps isolate your lower lats.

Action: The first pull is with your shoulders. In other words, pull your shoulders down before you even bend your arms. Next, hoist your body up until your chin is just above the bar. At the top, make sure your shoulders are pressed down. Pull your elbows in to your sides at the same time.

Performance Points: A wide grip on this exercise will help build the upper lats and rhomboids.

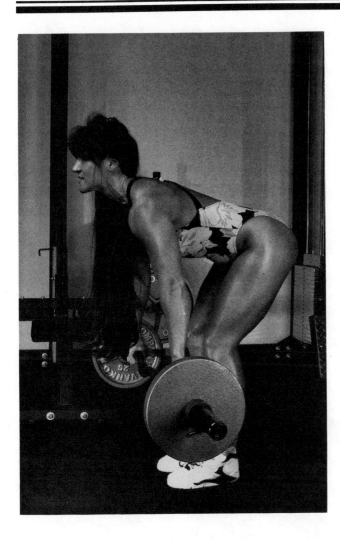
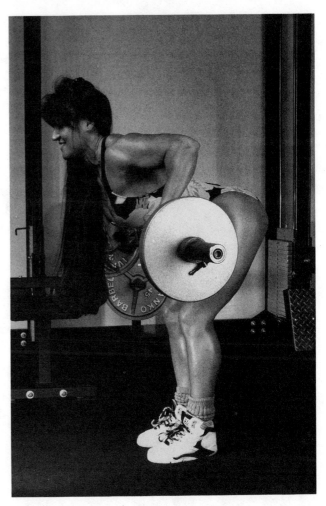

Bent-over Rows

Muscles Worked: Bent-over rows work the rhomboid muscles of the midback, with secondary emphasis on the lats, rear deltoid, biceps, forearms, and teres major and minor (two muscles located near the rear shoulders and upper arm in the upper back).

Start: To perform this exercise correctly, take a wide grip on the barbell (a close grip places too much emphasis on the arms). Keep your back slightly arched throughout the movement and your shoulders back.

Action: Pull the bar up toward your pecs. Pinch your scapula (shoulder blades) at the top of the movement. Keep your back muscles tight and use the strength of your pecs to push the bar back down. Be sure to keep constant tension on the working muscles throughout the range of motion.

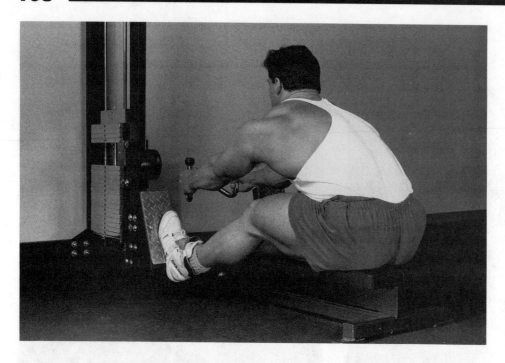

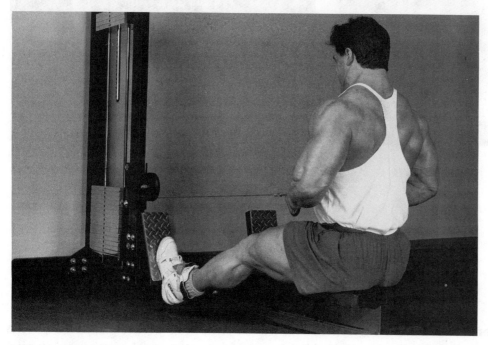

Seated Rows

Muscles Worked: **This exercise builds the lats and upper back.**

Start: **Lean forward and make the initial pull with your shoulders. Pull the handle toward your midsection, keeping your shoulders down.**

Action: **At the top of the exercise, sit straight up, push your chest out, and pinch your scapula together. Return slowly to the starting position, stretching forward at the bottom of the movement.**

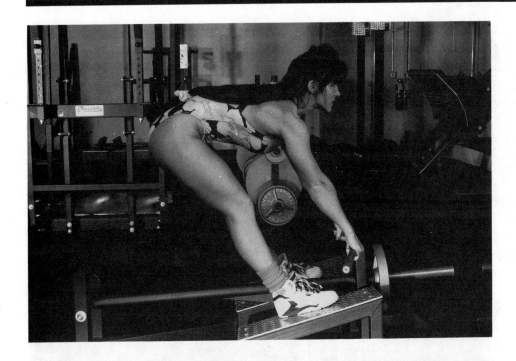

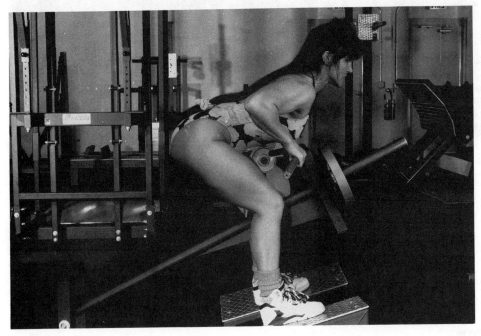

T-Bar Rows

Muscles Worked: This is an excellent exercise for building the rhomboids, lats, and teres.

Start: Grip the bar, keeping your back slightly arched. Press your shoulders back and keep them in this position throughout the exercise.

Action: Pull the bar in toward your torso. Squeeze your rhomboids and lower lats in the contracted position. Lower slowly to the starting position, using the strength of your pectoral muscles and front delts. Keep constant tension on the muscles throughout the entire range of motion.

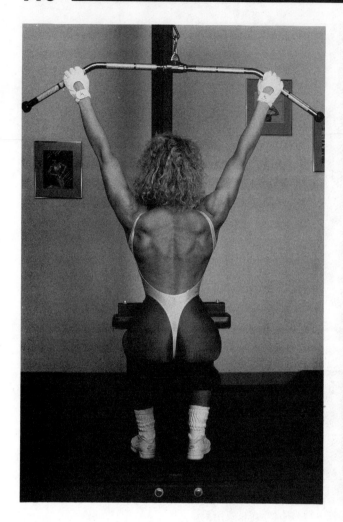 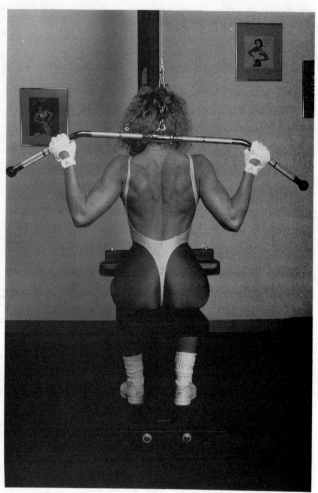

Behind-the-Neck Pulldowns

Muscles Worked: This exercise builds the upper lats and rhomboids.

Start: Take a wide overhand grip on the bar. As you begin the exercise, pull your shoulders down.

Action: Pull the bar down behind you, press your elbows back, and arch your back. Stay tight throughout the exercise.

Performance Points: To work your lower lats with this exercise, pump them before letting the bar return to the start position.

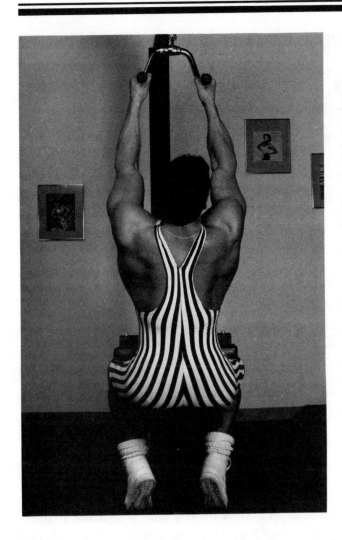 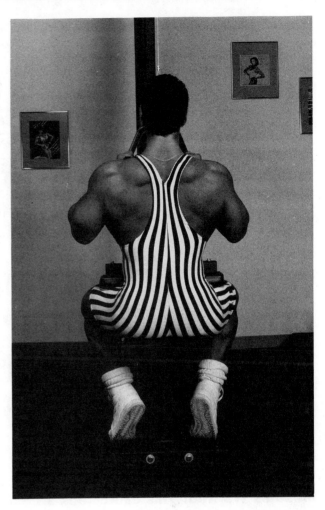

Front Lat Pulldowns

Muscles Worked: Front lat pulldowns emphasize your lower lats.

Start: Take a narrow grip on the bar. As you begin the exercise, pull your shoulders down and keep them in this position throughout the exercise. Do not lean back during the exercise.

Action: As you pull the bar down, bring your elbows in close to your sides. Keep everything tight.

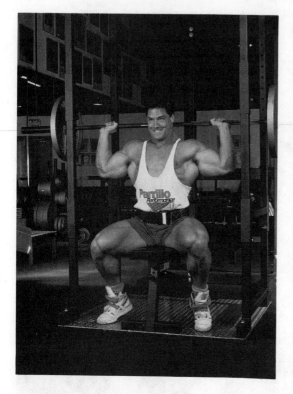
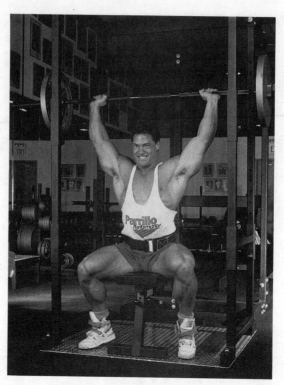

SHOULDER EXERCISES

Behind-the-Neck Press

Muscles Worked: This exercise is an excellent mass builder for the shoulder region because it stresses all three heads of the deltoid as well as the trapezius, a kite-shaped muscle that starts at the base of the neck and goes to the midback.

Start: Take a seated position and a wide grip on the barbell. Drop your shoulders and flex your lats.

Action: Press the weight upward, straightening your elbows. As you lock out, press your hips forward while tightening your abs. Then push the weight back slightly, but without arching your back. This entire action isolates your delts. All the emphasis is right on your shoulders. You'll really feel it!

Performance Points: The most common technique error I see with this exercise is excessive arching of the back. Bodybuilders arch in this manner so they can better lift and maneuver heavier weights to the overhead position. This leads to poor shoulder flexibility, a problem even the most well-developed bodybuilders have.

I have often been asked about the effectiveness of front presses versus behind-the-neck presses. Personally, I prefer behind-the-neck presses. With front presses, there is an even greater tendency to arch backwards, limiting the efficiency of the movement. My recommendation is to stick to behind-the-neck presses. Not only will these widen your shoulder and pectoral carriage when performed correctly, they will also build the trapezius. Many bodybuilders have shallow backs because they have not built their lower trapezius, which supports the musculature of the back. Perform behind-the-neck presses correctly, and you'll build bigger traps and a larger back overall.

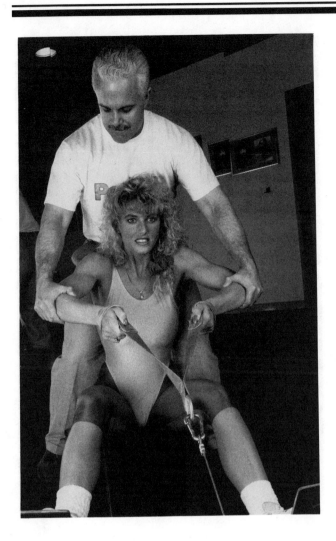 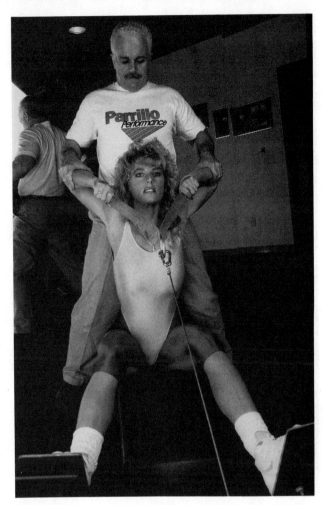

Shoulder Rows

Muscles Worked: For maximum stress on the delts, this exercise is best performed using a wrist strap attachment.

Start: Slip your hands through the loops of the straps and twist both your elbows and the palms of your hands outward.

Action: With assistance from your workout partner, pull your elbows back as far as possible. Keep your shoulders down. As you descend, rotate your arms so that your palms face inward. In a slow, controlled fashion, move your arms into a "crab pose" position and return to start.

Performance Points: With this exercise, you can go as heavy as possible with as many reps as possible—as long as your partner assists you.

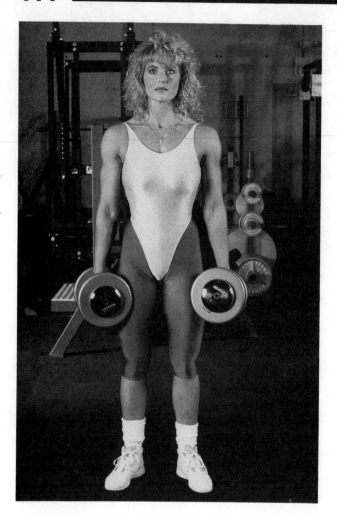 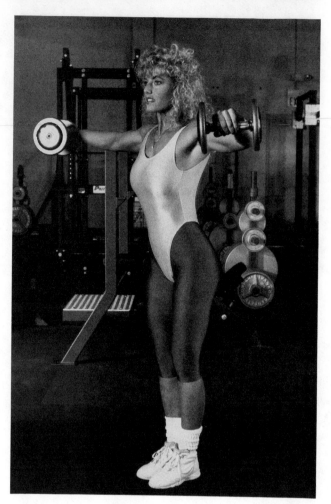

Lateral Raises

Muscles Worked: Lateral raises stress the deltoids.

Start: Take a dumbbell in each hand and hold them at the sides of your body.

Action: Raise the dumbbells upward, keeping your elbows rotated back. At the top of the exercise, lower your shoulders. Together, the elbow and shoulder positions keep the stress firmly on your deltoids.

Performance Points: An alternative to the lateral raise is the front raise, in which the dumbbells (or a barbell) is lifted out in front of your body. This variation stresses the front delts.

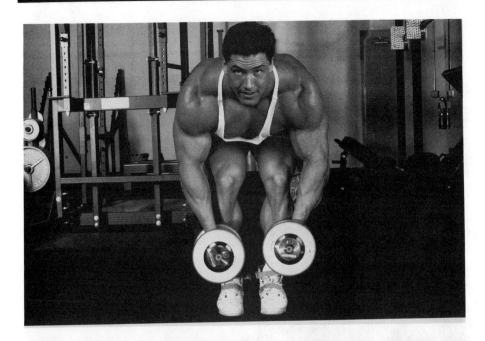

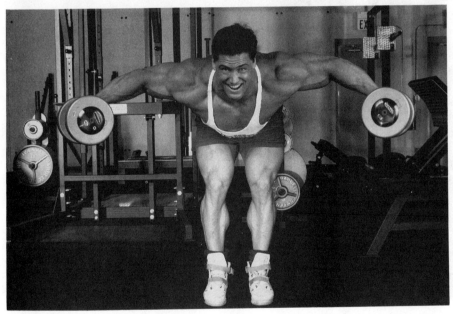

Bent-over Lateral Raises

Muscles Worked: This is an excellent isolation movement for the rear delts.

Start: Holding two dumbbells, bend over so that your upper body is parallel to the floor.

Action: Using your rear delts and not your rhomboids, lift the weight up from your sides and extend your arms. Squeeze your rear delts in the contracted position. Lower slowly back to start, using the strength of your muscles and not the momentum of the weight. Stay tight throughout the exercise.

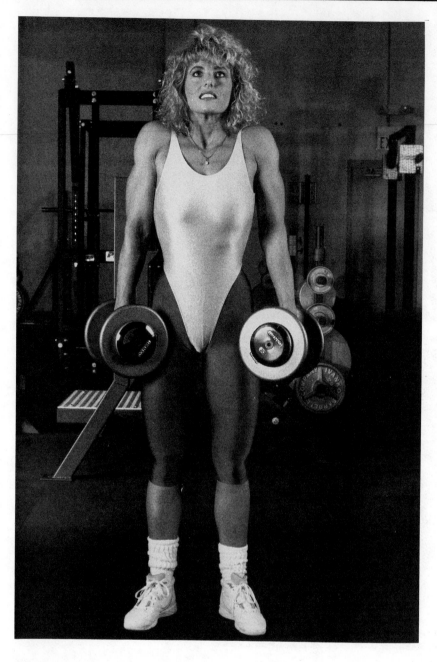

Shrugs

Muscles Worked: **This exercise directly stresses the trapezius.**

Start: **Take a dumbbell in each hand and hold them at your side.**

Action: **Lift the weight, using the strength of your traps. Be sure to squeeze your traps hard at the top of the movement.**

Performance Points: **Many bodybuilders like to include shrugs in their routines. But if you're doing squats, deadlifts, and heavy behind-the-neck presses, you may not need to add shrugs to your routine—unless your traps lag in development. You can also perform shrugs with a barbell.**

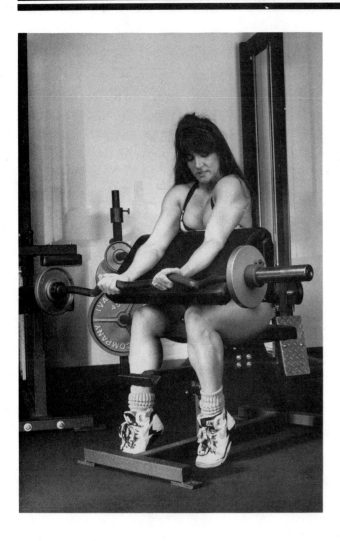 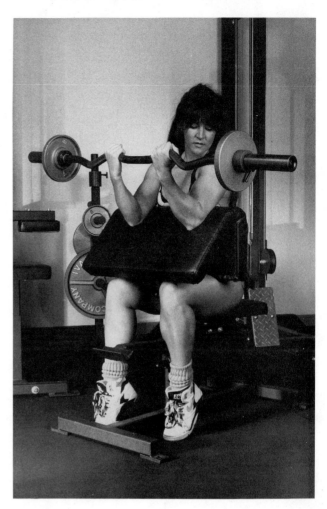

Preacher Curls

Muscles Worked: Preacher curls emphasize the biceps, with secondary stress on the forearm.

Start: Preacher curls can be performed with a barbell, dumbbells, or a cable handle attached to a weight stack. Take the bar and place your upper arms just against the upper end of the preacher curl bench.

Action: Lift the weight upward in an arc, keeping constant tension on the muscles. At the top of the exercise, pull your elbows together. This action isolates the biceps for a deep burn. As you return to the start position, use the strength of your triceps to pull the weight back into the start position.

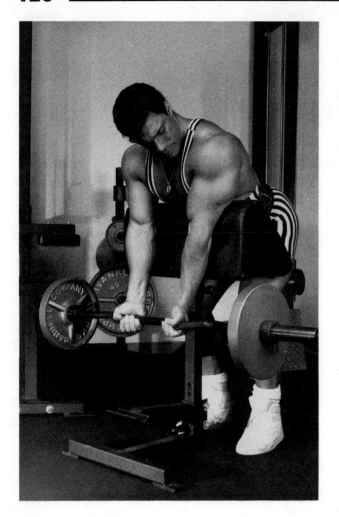 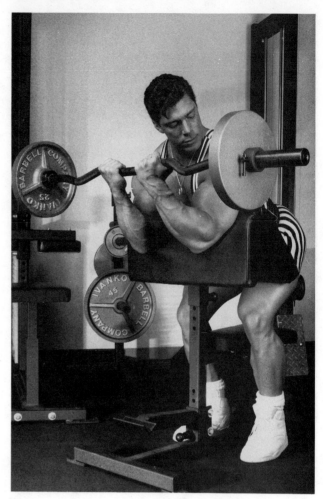

Spider Curls

Muscles Worked: **An alternative to the preacher curl, this exercise also works the biceps.**

Start: **The difference between the two exercises is that in the spider curl, you lean over the bench so that your arms point straight down as you begin the exercise. In this position, your torso is nearly parallel to the floor.**

Action: **Curl up, keeping your arms tight. Squeeze hard in the contracted position. Then lower the weight slowly, using the strength of your triceps.**

Performance Points: **An excellent isolation exercise for biceps, spider curls are more difficult to do than preacher curls. Add them to your arm routine for extra intensity.**

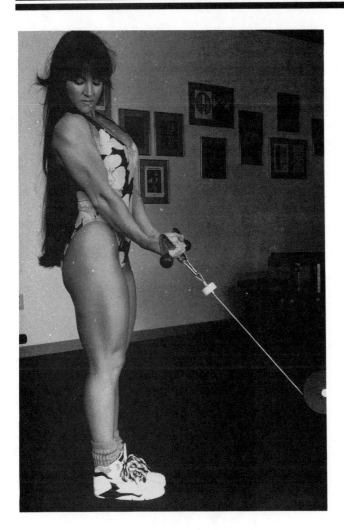 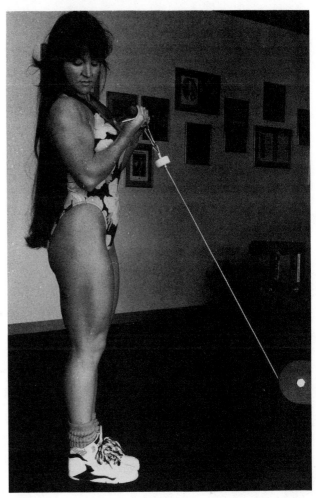

Cable Curls

Muscles Worked: **This is an excellent muscle-shaping movement for the biceps.**

Start: **Grasp a low pulley with one hand with your palm facing forward and arm pressed close to your side.**

Action: **Flex your arm at the elbow, curling up toward your chest. Keep constant tension on the working muscles. Lower to the start position, using the strength of your triceps. Work the other arm with an equal number of reps.**

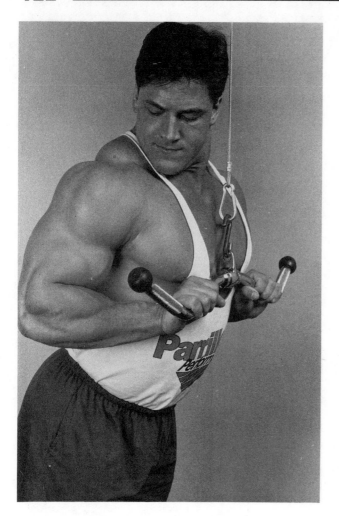 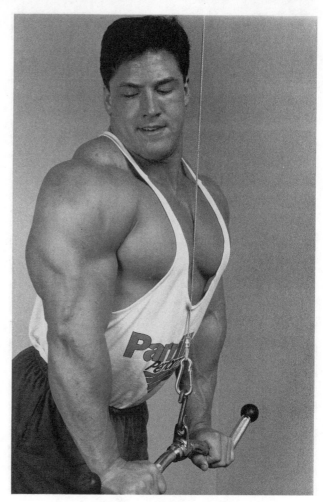

Triceps Pressdown

Muscles Worked: **This is an excellent exercise for building the triceps muscle of the upper arm.**

Start: **Take a narrow overgrip on the bar. Keep your upper arms and elbows pressed close to the sides of your body.**

Action: **Push down to a fully locked-out position. Keep your arms and elbows in this position throughout the range of motion. Stay tight and use the strength of your biceps to return the weight to the start position.**

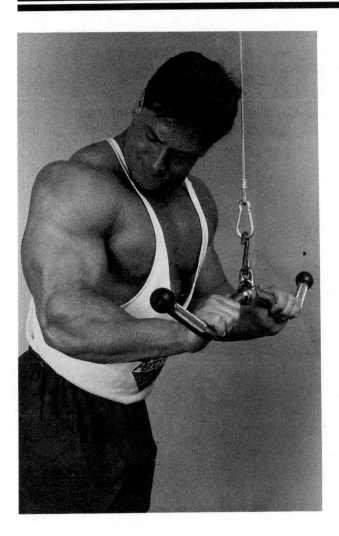 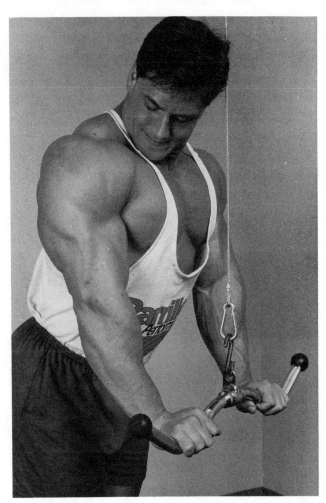

Variation: Another way to perform the triceps pressdown is what I call "the cheating method." This version builds the belly (the third head of the triceps). To begin, keep your elbows angled out away from your body as you push through the exercise. Guide the bar straight up to your lower pec. Rely on the strength of your biceps to pull the weight to the start position. Stay tight throughout the exercise.

Performance Points: Bodybuilders typically have well-developed heads on their triceps because they perform their exercises very strictly. Powerlifters, on the other hand, have huge triceps because they cheat their exercises. To get the best of both worlds, use both the strict and the cheating methods in your arm routines.

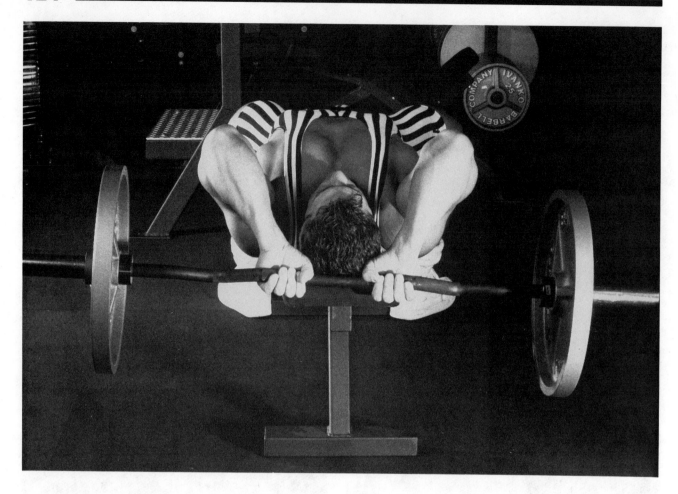

Conventional Triceps Extension

Muscles Worked: This exercise directly stresses the triceps.

Start: Lie back on a flat bench. Begin with a straight or an EZ-curl bar extended overhead. Lower the bar to the top of the bench.

Action: Press the bar up, allowing it to travel in an arc to an overhead position.

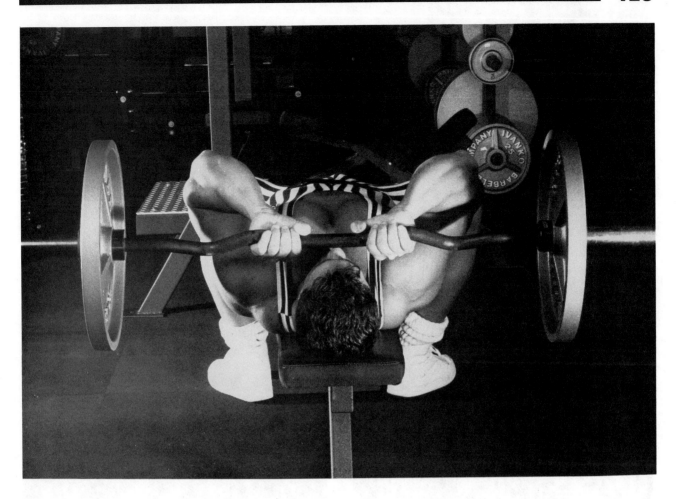

Skull Crushers

Muscles Worked: This exercise is an effective alternative to conventional triceps extensions, especially if you want to stress the long head of your triceps.

Start: Lie back on a flat bench. Begin with a straight or an **EZ-curl** bar extended in an overhead position. Bend your elbows to lower the bar just to your chin, not to your forehead or the top of the bench.

Action: Press back up. Make sure the bar moves up and down in a straight line, rather than in an arc as you would do with strict triceps extensions.

Performance Points: Let your elbows come out as you perform the exercise. Be sure to stay strict and tight. Always use the strength of your biceps to lower the weight.

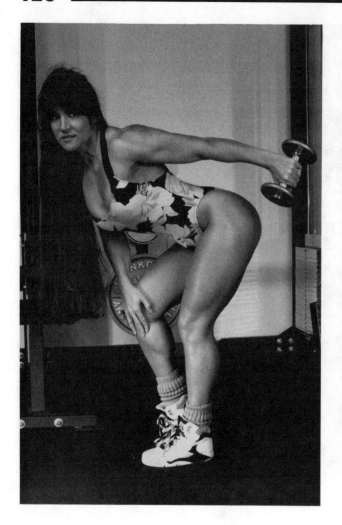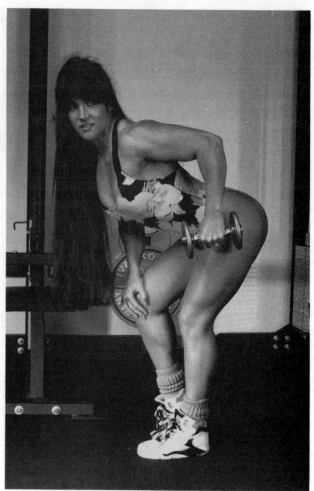

Triceps Kickback

Muscles Worked: **This is an excellent isolation movement for the triceps.**

Start: **Holding a dumbbell in one hand, bend over so that your upper body is parallel to the floor. Extend your arm straight out behind you, keeping your elbow as high as you can. Drop your shoulders.**

Action: **Flex at the elbow, bringing the weight toward the side of your chest. Squeeze as tightly as possible in the contracted position.**

Performance Points: **Stay tight throughout the range of motion. Use the strength of your biceps to pull your arm back to the starting position.**

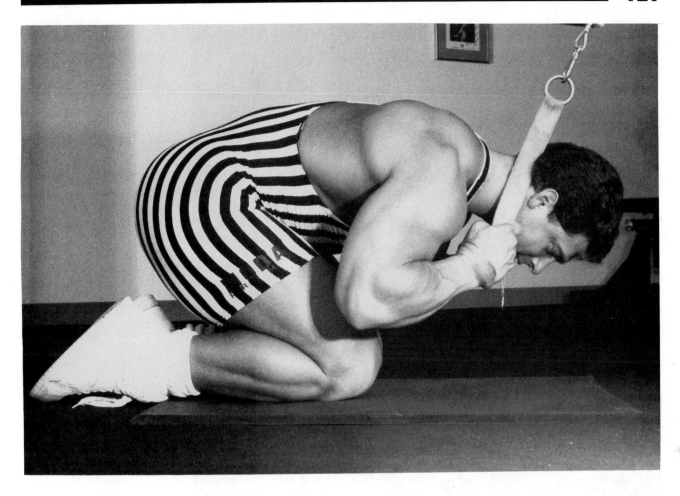

ABDOMINAL EXERCISES

Cable Crunches

Muscles Worked: This is a good, all-around exercise for the upper and lower abdominals.

Start: Grasp the rope or handle of a high pulley machine. Tuck your pelvic girdle in and forward as you perform the movement. Unless you adopt this position, your lower abs will go unworked.

Action: Crunch down, using the strength of your ab muscles. Keep these muscles completely tensed as you perform the exercise.

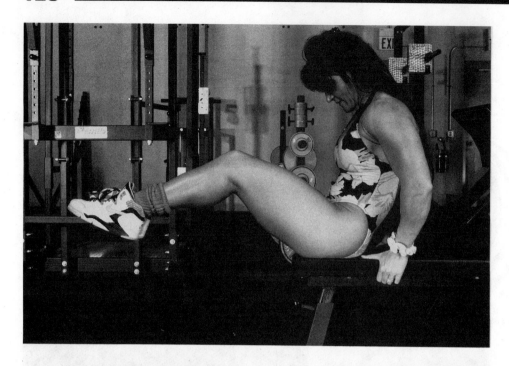

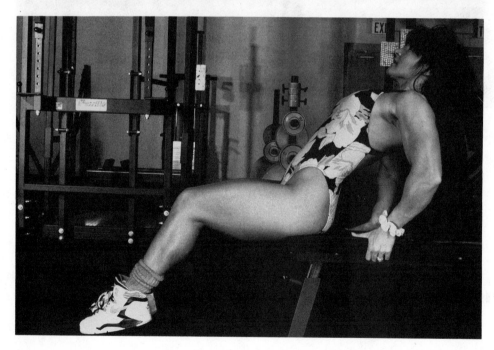

Leg Lifts

Muscles Worked: **This movement places direct stress on the lower abs.**

Start: **Sit at the edge of a bench and extend your legs out in front of you, stretching your torso. As you extend your legs, arch your back.**

Action: **Pull your knees in toward your chest, and then bow your back. Crunch and squeeze your abs. Do not pivot at the hip joint.**

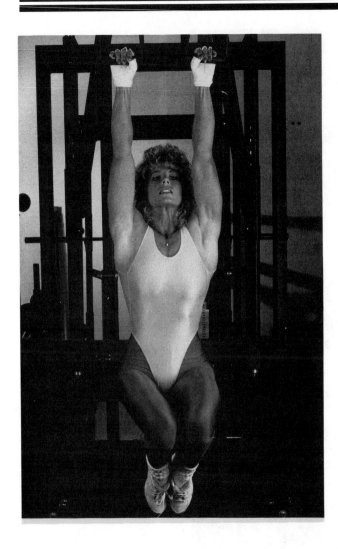 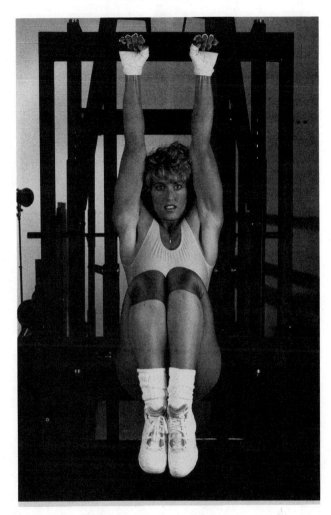

Hanging Leg Raises

Muscles Worked: Hanging leg raises stress the serratus, a group of several muscles located between the ribs and shoulder blade.

Start: Take a medium grip on a chinning bar. Bend your knees and hold them out in front of you.

Action: Crunch your midsection. Then twist slightly to one side and then to the other. Keep your abs tight. Squeeze your abs and serratus without moving your hip joint.

Performance Points: Many bodybuilders train their abs under the misguided notion that they should work their obliques, a group of muscles covering the sides of the midsection. Unless you want a thick, unflattering waist, do not exercise your obliques. Concentrate on the serratus muscles. The hanging leg raise is the best exercise for developing these muscles.

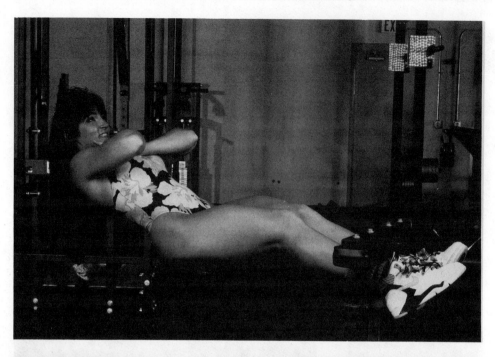

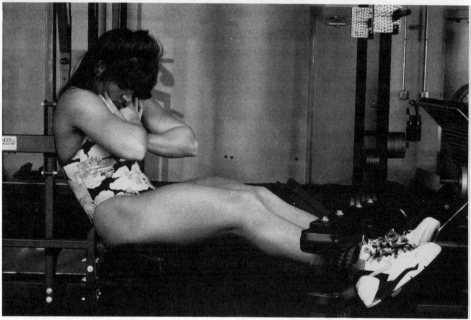

Roman Chair Sit-up

Muscles Worked: An alternative to cable crunches, this exercise also works the upper and lower abs.

Start: Sit in the Roman chair and lean back to a fully extended position. Your torso should be below parallel to the floor. As you lean back, get a good stretch in your abdominals.

Action: Using the strength of your ab muscles, crunch tightly to bring your torso forward. Keep your abdominal muscles very tight as you lean back and crunch forward.

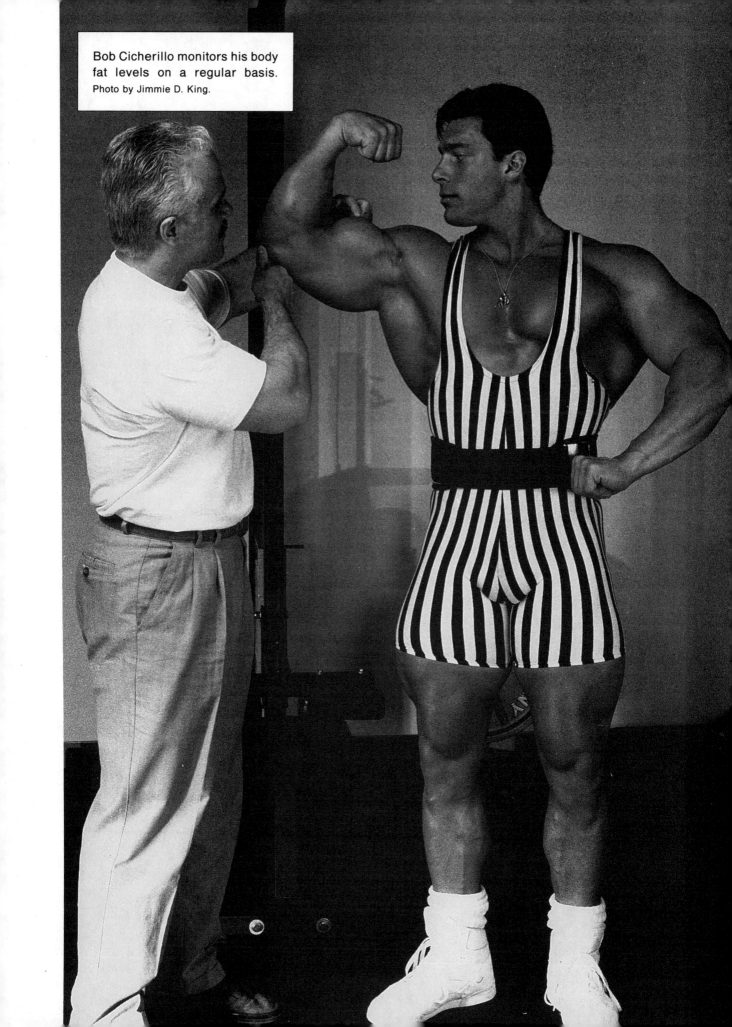

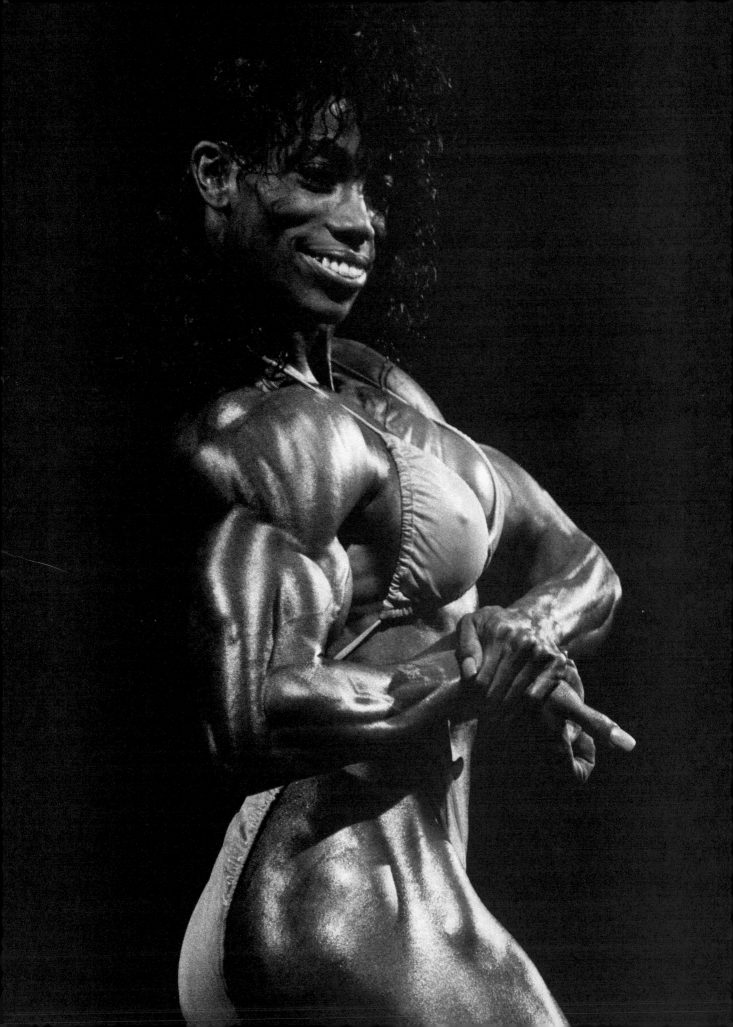

NINE
FASCIAL STRETCHING: OPEN UP YOUR GROWTH ZONE

Bigger muscles, deeper separations, greater strength—these can all be achieved by a specialized training technique I developed just for bodybuilders. It's called "fascial stretching," and its effect on the physique is nothing short of amazing.

Understanding the technique of fascial stretching starts with some basic anatomy involving the fascia. The fascia is one of six internal tissues of the body, along with muscles, tendons, bones, joints, and ligaments. It is a thick, fibrous sheet that envelops individual muscles and groups of muscles and, like a divider, separates their layers and groupings. The fascia encloses other structures too, including tendons, joints, blood vessels, nerves, and organs. In fact, there are more than 50 types of fascia tissue throughout the body.

Think of the fascia as a shock absorber for the tissues it surrounds, protecting them from blows of athletics or the stresses of training. And what a protector it is: On the molecular level, fascia tissue is stronger than structural steel.

Fascial stretching is a method of stretching this tissue to stimulate growth, improve muscular size, shape, separation, and strength. By stretching the fascia, you give the muscle underneath more room to grow, thus opening up a whole new "growth zone."

To get these results, you must stretch the fascia between each exercise set—when the muscles are fully pumped. The pump itself has a pre-stretch effect on the fascia. Fascial stretching, combined with a pump, stretches the fascia to its limit.

You can improve your pump—and therefore your ability to stretch the fascia—by adhering to my nutritional recommendations. A high-calorie, nutrient-dense diet loads more glycogen into the muscles. This glycogen-load leads to huge pumps.

In women's bodybuilding, the exceptional Lenda Murray is the shape of things to come. Photo by J.M. Manion.

With fascial stretching, your strength can increase by as much as 20 percent—an increase related to a phenomenon known as the golgi tendon reflex (GTR) threshold. This describes a point at which your muscles shut down when tendons become overstretched by heavy weight.

With a high GTR threshold, you can handle heavier weights and a greater number of reps—an ability ultimately resulting in greater gains. One way to increase your GTR threshold is with regular fascial stretching. It conditions your muscles and connective tissue to withstand ever-increasing weight and reps.

The benefits of fascial stretching don't end with muscle size and strength. Stretching makes your body more flexible, giving your muscles and the joints they connect greater range of motion. A supple, flexible physique is less susceptible to injuries because it can better withstand physical stresses. Stretching also helps prevent muscle soreness and promotes better recovery.

In addition, stretching loosens tight muscles, which tend to trap lactic acid, a waste product that accumulates in muscle cells during hard training. When lactic acid builds up, muscular fatigue is the result. Stretching helps release lactic acid from muscle cells into the bloodstream so that it does not interfere with muscular contraction. This loosening effect of stretching also helps you breathe better during workouts, and this increases your oxygen utilization for improved energy levels.

Fascial stretching is by no means the gentle, touch-your-toes type of exercise you might associate with conventional stretching. Instead, it is forceful enough to elicit some contorted grimaces from even the most hard-core bodybuilders.

Nor are the stretching exercises themselves conventional. I have developed 28 special fascial-stretching exercises for specific parts of the body. As the stretch begins, the body part being trained is guided into position, stretched past the point of pain, and then held in that position for about 10 seconds. You should exhale and relax as you go into the stretch. Never hold your breath, either.

There are two methods of stretching—the self-stretches and the partner-assisted stretches. The self-stretches are a good starting point, particularly if you have never stretched before or do not train with a partner. But to continue to make significant muscular gains, you need to do the partner-assisted stretches—and do them every workout. You can get a much deeper, harder stretch by working with a partner.

Workout quality—as measured by intensity and effectiveness—is enhanced by including fascial stretching. The reason is: A portion of the typical rest period between sets is devoted to stretching exercises, which alone are intense and energy-demanding. Fascial stretching will not prolong your workouts but instead will make them much more productive.

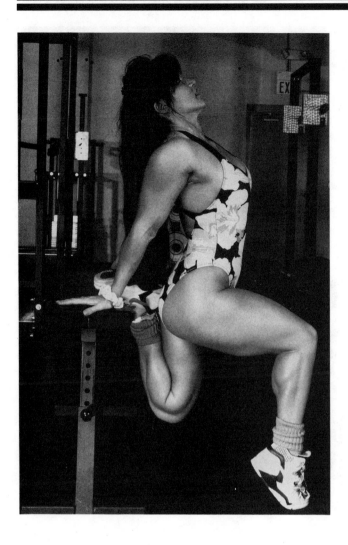

LEG FASCIAL STRETCHES

Quad Stretch

Start: Stand next to a bench or other piece of sturdy gym equipment. Bend your right knee. Holding your right ankle, bring your bent leg behind you. Position your ankle so that your instep is secured against the equipment. For balance, hold on to the equipment.

Stretch: Press your right heel to your glute while pushing your quad down and back. Hold for 10 seconds, then release. Repeat with the left quad.

Variation: To stretch your upper quad, press your leg down first. Then push your heel to your glute.

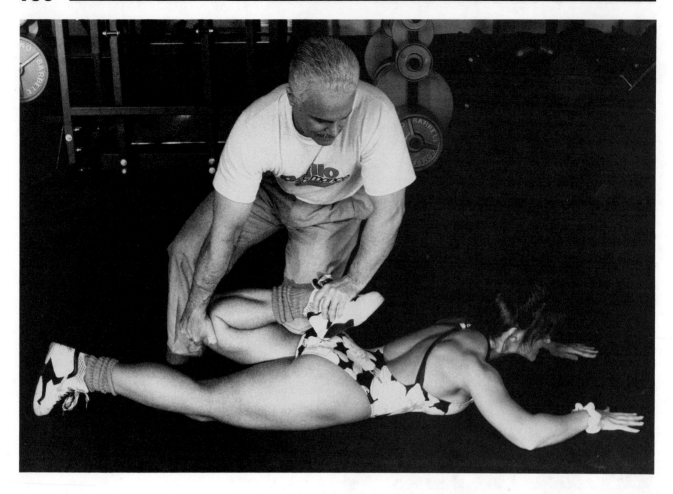

Quad Stretch/Partner-Assisted

Start: **Like most of these stretches, this one will feel painful at first. The pain merely indicates that your quads are very tight. Many of the bodybuilders I stretch can barely get their knees off the floor. After a few workouts, however, I can lift their quads up 45 degrees or more.**

To begin, lie on your stomach. Then bend your elbows and rest your head on your forearms. Bend your left leg up so that your heel touches your glutes.

Stretch: **Your partner presses down on your left ankle while pulling your bent leg upward with his right hand, as illustrated. This position is held for 10 seconds. You should feel an intense stretch in your quad. Repeat with the opposite leg.**

Variation: **To stretch a higher portion of your quad, have your partner place his knee at your glute/hamstring tie-in. He pulls your knee up, then pushes your heel down to your glute.**

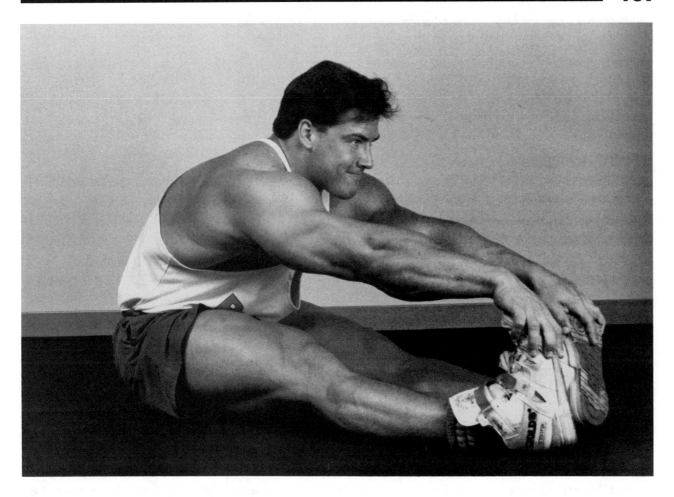

Forward Hamstring Stretch

Start: **This movement stretches the hamstring and strengthens the lower back, making it an excellent stretch for people with lower-back problems. To begin, sit with your legs extended straight out in front of you. Lean forward and clasp the tops of your feet. Make sure your knees are locked out tightly.**

Stretch: **Lean forward, arching your back as hard as you can, as illustrated. Pull the tops of your feet toward you. Stretch hard. Hold for a count of 10 before releasing.**

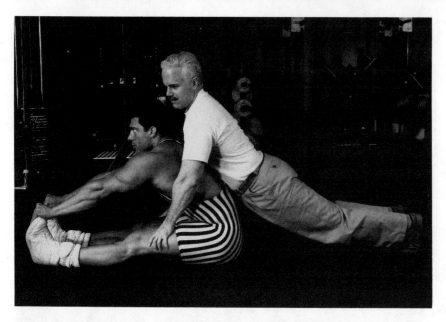

Forward Hamstring Stretch/Partner-Assisted

Start: Sit on the floor with your legs extended straight out and pressed together. Lean forward and clasp the balls of your feet with your hands and pull back. Try to keep the backs of your knees flat on the floor. Your partner is positioned directly behind you so that his stomach is pressed against your lower back.

Stretch: As your partner presses forward, you should feel a strong stretch in your hamstrings and gastrocnemius muscles. The stretched position is held for a count of 10.

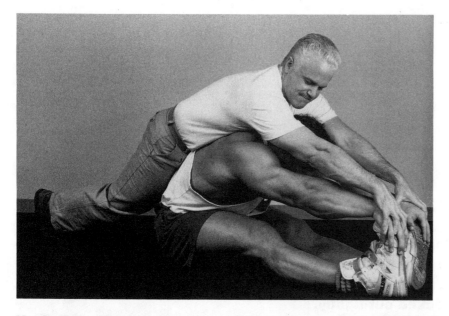

Variation: Your partner can also grab your feet with his hands to further stretch your hamstrings and gastrocnemius. A word of caution: Make sure he doesn't push against your upper back.

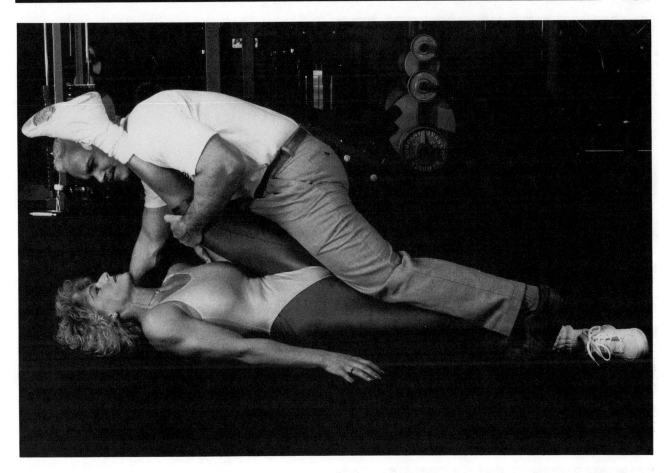

Hamstring Stretch/Partner-Assisted

Start: Lie on your back and extend your left leg so that it is perpendicular to the floor. Facing you in a lunge position, your partner positions himself so that his left knee is pressed down on your right thigh to secure your hip. Your left ankle is against his left shoulder, as illustrated. He clasps his hands over your left knee.

Stretch: Your partner then lunges forward, pushing your raised leg toward your head. This motion stretches your hamstring. The stretched position is held for 10 seconds. Repeat with the right leg.

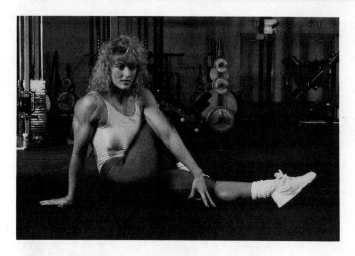

Hip Stretch

Start: Sit on the floor with your legs extended out in front of you. Bend your right leg and cross it over your left leg. Place your elbow as low on your leg as you can.

Stretch: Rotate your upper body as far to the right as you can. Turn your shoulders around, pushing your knee over. Balance yourself with your hands. Hold for 10 seconds, then release. Repeat the stretch with your left leg.

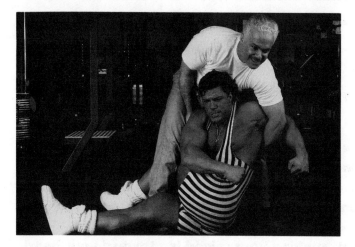

Hip Stretch/Partner-Assisted

Start: Sit on the floor with your legs extended straight out in front of you. Bend and lift your left leg up. Cross it over your right leg. With his right leg, your partner steps through the triangle created by the position of your legs, anchoring your bent leg in position, as illustrated. He then loops his arms under your shoulders and grabs the inside of his left knee with his left hand.

Stretch: Your partner twists your body to the left, as he straightens his left leg, pushes your right shoulder forward, and pulls your left shoulder back. This action really stretches your hip. Repeat with the other side of the body.

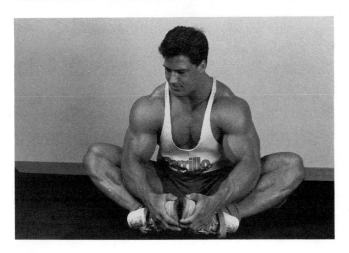

Butterfly

Start: **This movement stretches your inner thighs and hips. Sit on the floor with your knees bent and the bottoms of your feet pressed together.**

Stretch: **With your back arched, move your upper body toward the floor while pressing your inner thighs down with your forearms. Hold for a count of 10.**

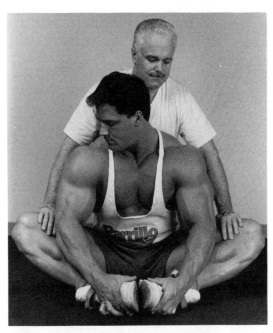

Butterfly/Partner-Assisted

Start: **Sit on the floor, bend your knees out, and place the bottoms of your feet together. Kneeling behind you, your partner presses his stomach against your lower back and places his hands on the inner portion of your knees.**

Stretch: **Lean forward slightly, bringing your upper body toward the floor. Your partner assists the stretch by pushing forward with his stomach against your lower back and by pushing down on your knees. The stretched position is held for 10 seconds.**

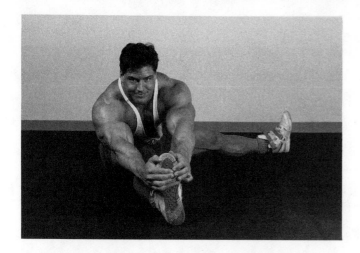

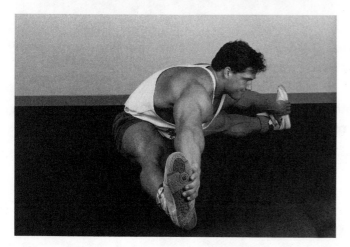

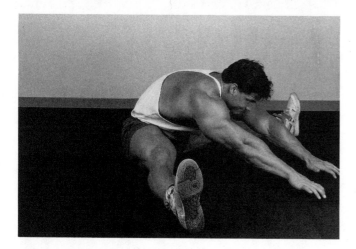

Inner-Thigh Stretches

Start: Sit on the floor with your legs spread wide apart.

Stretch: Reach over your right leg and grasp your right foot with both hands. Lean toward your foot and stretch hard. In the next stretch, grasp your feet with your hands and lean forward toward the floor. In the final stretch, lean forward with your hands outstretched in front of you. Push your body toward the floor.

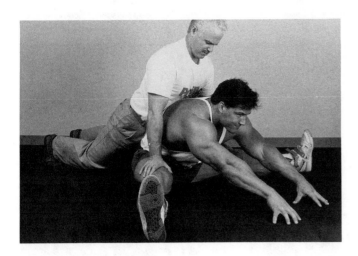

Forward Inner-Thigh/Hamstring Stretch/Partner-Assisted

Start: Sit on the floor with your legs spread wide apart. Your partner is positioned directly behind you, with his stomach pressed against your lower back and his hands above your knees.

Stretch: Your partner presses your upper body toward the floor as you "walk" forward with your hands as far as you can. Hold for a count of 10, then release. For a deeper stretch, your partner can put his hands under your legs and pull too.

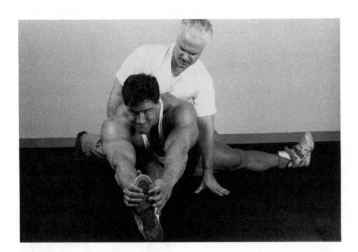

Inner-Thigh Stretch to the Side/Partner-Assisted

Start: Sit on the floor and spread your legs. Your partner presses his stomach against your lower back and places his hands on your quads.

Stretch: Lean forward toward your right foot. Grab your toes and pull toward you, as illustrated. As you stretch forward, your partner presses against your lower back. Hold the stretched position for 10 seconds, then repeat on the other side. Have your partner grasp underneath your leg for a deeper, more intense stretch.

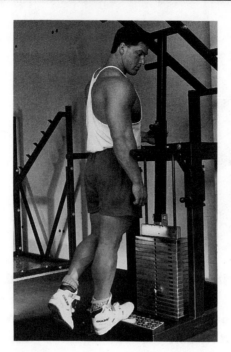
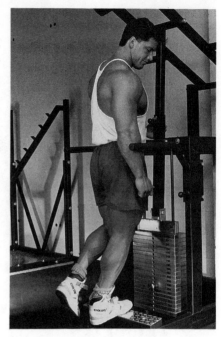

Calf Stretch

Start: With one foot, stand on a block of wood or elevated platform. For balance, hold on to a piece of equipment. Keep all your weight on the calf being stretched. To stretch your gastrocnemius, keep your knee locked. To stretch your soleus, keep it flexed. For an even greater stretch, use a standing calf machine. Allow the weight of the machine to push you down for a deep stretch.

Stretch: Rise up on the ball of your foot, lifting your heel as high as you can. Then lower your heel toward the floor, obtaining a deep stretch as you press down. Repeat the stretch with your other leg.

CHEST FASCIAL STRETCHES

Medium Grip Skin-the-Cat

Start: Skin-the-cat is a gymnastics-type movement that requires a great deal of practice. To stretch the pecs, it should be performed with a medium grip. To begin, take an overhand grip on the pull-up bar. Bend your knees and pull yourself up.

Stretch: Next invert your body, pulling your feet in through the opening created by your hands. Then rotate around to a hanging position, as illustrated. On your way down, tuck your knees to your chest. At the completion of the movement, point your toes and try to touch the floor. Your partner may assist you by helping you through the movement. The entire stretch should be performed slowly, with complete muscular control.

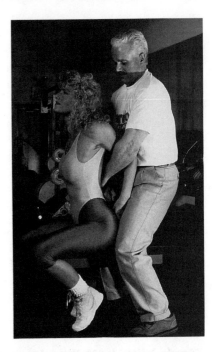

Pec Stretch/Partner-Assisted

Start: This stretch can be performed from a seated or standing position. To begin, press your shoulders and arms back. Standing behind you, your partner threads his arms through yours so that his elbows meet your elbows. Your partner clasps his wrist with one hand. Be sure to push your chest out.

Stretch: Arch your back as your partner pulls your arms together, straightening his arms as he pulls back. The stretch should be held for 10 seconds before releasing.

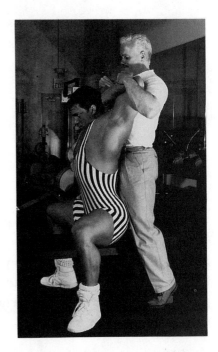

Pec/Shoulder Stretch/Partner-Assisted

Start: Seated on a bench, clasp your hands behind your neck. Point your elbows slightly upward toward the ceiling, as illustrated. From a standing position, your partner presses his stomach against your back.

Stretch: Holding your elbows, your partner stretches your upper arms up and back. The stretched position is held for 10 seconds.

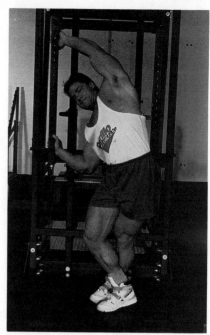

BACK FASCIAL STRETCHES

Lat Stretch

Start: With both hands, grasp a bar or piece of stationary equipment. Place all the weight on the left side of your body—the side that will be stretched first. Cross your right leg over your left leg and step forward so that all your weight is on your left foot.

Stretch: Lean away from the bar, forming a comma with your body. With your left hand, push your shoulders in and through, as illustrated. Hold this position for 10 seconds. Repeat with the other side of your body.

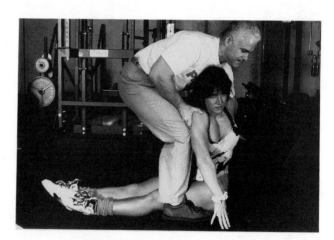

Twisting Stretch/Partner-Assisted

Start: Sit on the floor with your legs extended and together. Rotate your body slightly to the left. Facing you, your partner straddles your body just at your thighs. He then places his right hand and right knee under your shoulder. He also loops his left hand under your right shoulder.

Stretch: Straightening his left leg and bending his right leg, your partner then pulls up your torso, twisting your body further to the left. This position is held for 10 seconds. Repeat the stretch for the right side of your body.

Variation: To also stretch your rib cage, your partner lifts your arm up and back.

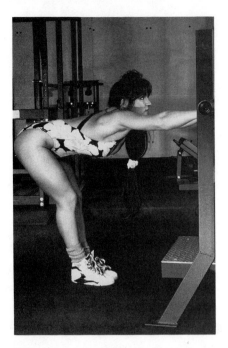

SHOULDER FASCIAL STRETCHES

Shoulder Stretch

Start: This stretch is performed at a bench-press rack with a bar. Bend at the waist and take a wide grip on the bar. Your upper body should be parallel to the floor, as illustrated.

Stretch: Flex your lats and lower your shoulders down toward the floor as far as you can. Keep your arms tightly locked. Hold this position for a count of 10, then release.

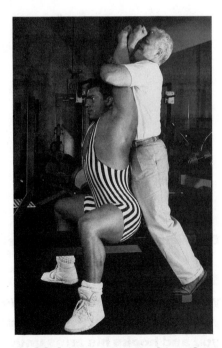

Shoulder/Rhomboid Stretch/Partner-Assisted

Start: Take a seated position. Extend and raise your arms as high as you can, keeping them straight. Press your wrists together. Standing behind you, your partner wraps his arms around your upper arms.

Stretch: Your partner then pushes down, stretching your entire delt area.

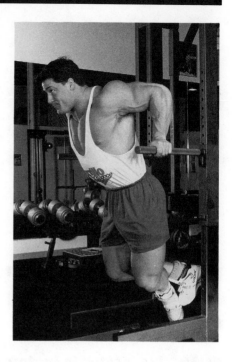

Delt Stretch with Dip Bars

Start: Grasp the dip bars with your palms facing inward.

Stretch: Keeping your knees bent, lower yourself as far down as you can. Press your elbows back. Hold the descended position for 10 seconds, then release.

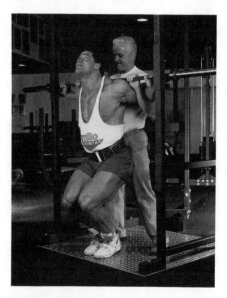

Delt/Upper-Pec Stretch/Partner-Assisted

Start: As if to perform a squat, position yourself at the barbell so that the bar is across your shoulders and behind your neck. The bar should be as far down on your back as possible. Lean forward slightly and point your elbows up. Your partner stands behind you and hooks his arms underneath your forearms. He places his hands on the bar just inside and next to your hands.

Stretch: With the strength of his upper body, your partner pushes your hips forward and your elbows up. Held for 10 seconds, this movement completely stretches and loosens your deltoids and pecs.

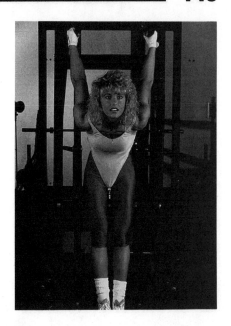

Narrow Grip Skin-the-Cat

Start: **To stretch the delts, skin-the-cats should be performed with a narrow grip. To begin, take an overhand grip on the pull-up bar. Bend your knees and pull yourself up.**

Stretch: **Next invert your body, pulling your feet in through the opening created by your hands. Then rotate around to a hanging position, as illustrated. On your way down, tuck your knees to your chest. At the completion of the movement, point your toes and try to touch the floor. Remember to perform the movement slowly, with complete muscular control.**

ARM FASCIAL STRETCHES

Wide Grip Skin-the-Cat

Start: **Wide-grip skin-the-cats are excellent for stretching the biceps. Begin by taking an overhand grip on the pull-up bar. Bend your knees and pull yourself up.**

Stretch: **As you did with the previous skin-the-cat stretches, invert your body, pulling your feet in through the opening created by your hands. Then rotate around to a hanging position. On your way down, tuck your knees to your chest. At the completion of the movement, point your toes and try to touch the floor. Get help from your partner if necessary. Use total muscular control when performing the stretch.**

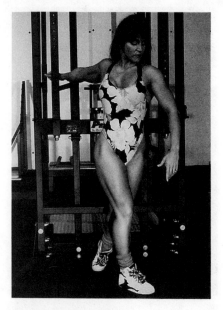

Biceps Stretch

Start: Stand at arm's length from the bar. Then grip the bar with your right hand, as illustrated.

Stretch: Rotate your torso as far to the left as you can. Hold for 10 seconds, then release. Repeat with the other arm.

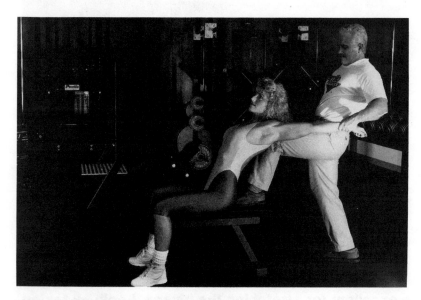

Biceps Stretch/Partner-Assisted

Start: Sit on a bench and lean back against your partner's lower leg. Extend your arms out behind you.

Stretch: Holding your wrists, your partner pulls your arms in and back. The stretched position is held for 10 seconds.

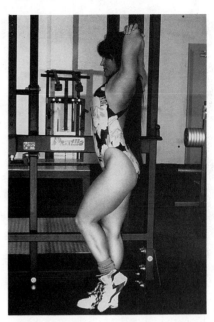

Triceps Stretch

Start: Place your back against a bar or piece of stationary equipment, as shown. Hold on to the equipment and push your shoulder up against the bar. This pushes your triceps up. Bend your arms behind your head and point your elbows up toward the ceiling. Grab your triceps with your other hand and pull it back. Bend your knees.

Stretch: To stretch your triceps, simply straighten your knees. Hold the stretched position for 10 seconds, then release.

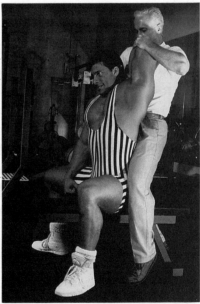

Triceps Stretch/Partner-Assisted

Start: Take a seated position. As if to perform a dumbbell triceps extension, bend your left arm and lift your elbow up so that it points to the ceiling. For leverage, your partner stands behind you with his stomach pressed against your back. With his left hand, your partner grasps your extended elbow. His right hand holds your wrist, which should be positioned at your rear delt.

Stretch: Your partner pushes your wrist against the back of your delt, while pressing your elbow up and back. This position is held for 10 seconds before being released. You should feel a deep stretch throughout the length of your triceps. Repeat with the other arm.

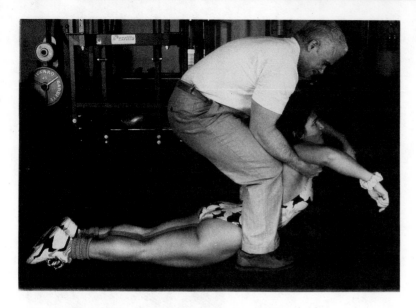

Abdominal Stretch/Partner-Assisted

Start: This stretch requires a great deal of caution to avoid unnecessary compression on the spine. Your partner should guide you through this stretch slowly and carefully, without any jerking motions. Lie on your stomach on the floor. Standing behind you, your partner straddles your body at your waistline, securing your hips with his feet and ankles. He hooks his arms under your shoulders.

Stretch: Your partner puts his knees together just at the center of your back. He lifts your torso up and then pulls up and back to a stretched position. This is held for 10 seconds. Your partner must be careful not to pull back and down. This action only places dangerous compression on the spine.

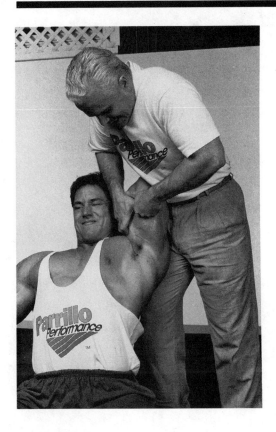

Fascial Planing

Once you have reached an advanced level in bodybuilding, you may want to try fascial planing—an ultra-advanced method of stretching the fascia through manual manipulation. Like fascial stretching, fascial planing stretches the fascia, maximizing the muscle's growth and separation potential.

Before the technique can be applied, however, you must attain a tremendous pump to first pre-stretch the fascia. Using the second joints of the knuckle, the manipulator (the training partner who performs the fascial planing) indents the fascia with a forceful pressure. Comparable to hard kneading, this indentation is made in a plane, moving from the muscle's insertion to its origin. This planing action should be performed 12 times. As with fascial stretching, the muscle being planed should next be posed.

This sequence of pumping the muscle, planing it, and posing it is performed three times at the end of the workout. The fascia tissue will then be stretched so much that the muscle underneath literally springs forth to fill the space yielded by the newly stretched fascia. This muscular response is dramatic. I once measured as much as two inches of growth in pro Ron Love's biceps after only a single session of fascia planing.

Bodybuilders admit that fascial planing is painful but nonetheless are willing to endure the temporary discomfort just to see a certain muscle respond. Fascial planing done once a week on a lagging body part forces muscular growth, deepens muscular separation, and makes the muscle look larger and fuller. A word of caution: this technique is designed for advanced, highly trained bodybuilders.

When combined with a nutrient-rich diet and intense training, both fascial stretching and fascial planing can take any advanced bodybuilder to a new level of physique perfection.

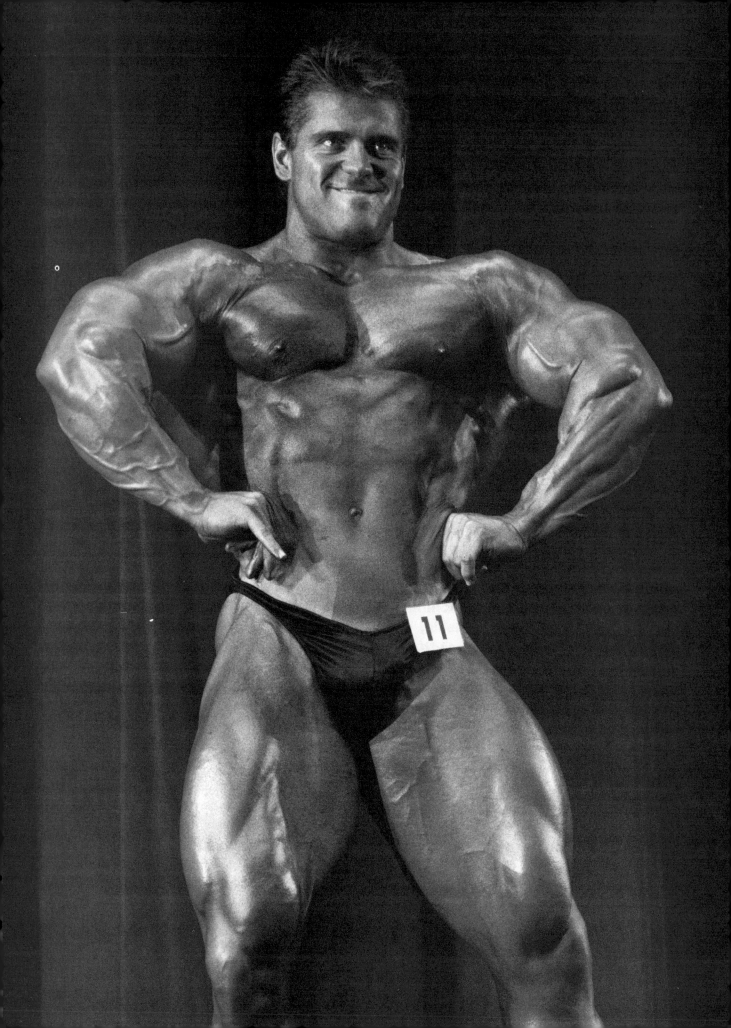

TEN WORKOUTS FOR MASS AND MUSCULARITY

The most effective training routines build two important components of muscular fitness: muscular density and cardiovascular density. Muscular density refers to the size and thickness of muscle fibers and is achieved by stressing the muscles with heavy weights. Heavy training stimulates growth of muscle fibers and develops and strengthens connective tissue.

To build muscular density, "pyramid" your sets, using low repetitions and heavy weights. Pyramiding, which is one of the most widely used training systems in bodybuilding, means increasing your poundages while decreasing your reps on each set.

To pyramid, begin with about eight to 12 reps on your first set. Add weight on each successive set while decreasing your reps. Perform between three to five sets per exercise, resting about two to five minutes between sets. The poundage should be so heavy on your last set that you can do no more than about three to

Eddie Robinson is undeniably a crowd favorite. Photo by J.M. Manion.

five reps. For even greater intensity, you may want to finish up with a heavy single (one rep) or a double (two reps) on your last set.

Of particular importance is that you avoid going to muscular failure (the point at which you can no longer complete a rep correctly) until you reach your heaviest set. That way, your energy reserves are not depleted. Nor is there any buildup of waste products in your muscles. Such a buildup would interfere with your ability to reach your maximum poundages.

As explained earlier, cardiovascular density describes the size and number of blood vessels in the muscle. These vessels carry oxygen and nutrients to the muscles and transport waste products away, and therefore are an important component in muscular growth and recovery.

Aerobic exercise is one way to building cardiovascular density; another is by high-repetition weight training in which you perform high-repetition (15 to 25)/ light weight sets after your pyramid sets. I call these sets "exhaustion sets."

Decrease your rest between sets to

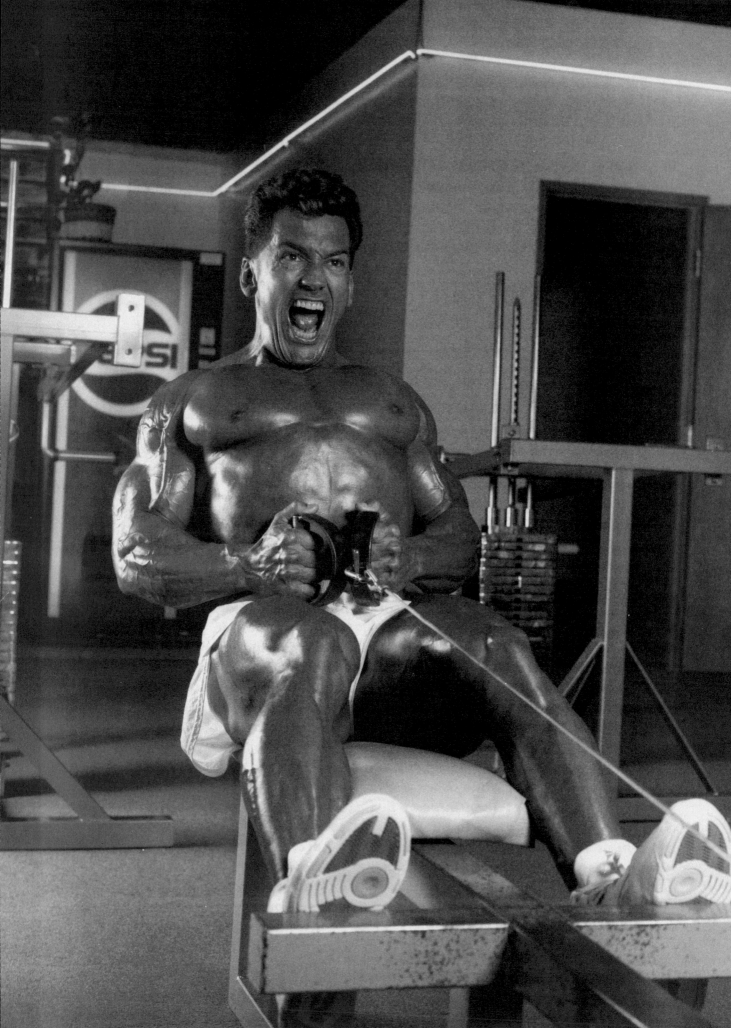

about 30 seconds to one minute. Rep out to muscular failure on every exhaustion set. Exhaustion sets improve muscular separation, giving your physique a well-defined, nicely shaped look.

FASCIAL STRETCHING

For maximum muscle growth, it's imperative that you stretch between sets. Use the stretching exercises covered in Chapter 9. If you're a competitive bodybuilder, pose the muscle group after stretching it. Posing increases muscular hardness, separation, and control. Combined with proper nutrition and hard training, stretching and flexing result in a quality look to the muscle that's impossible to achieve by any other technique.

HOW MANY SETS?

Bodybuilders always want to know how many total sets they should do for a particular exercise. In essence, you should work a muscle until you lose your pump. At that point, the muscle is out of glycogen. Further training only makes it harder for you to recover for your next workout.

The only time you should train past your pump is during pre-contest training. By training past your pump, you draw on fatty acids and amino acids as your energy source, since the muscle is depleted of glycogen. Extra body fat is burned as a result.

Pro Lee Labrada puts all-out effort into every rep. Photo by Jim Amentler.

USING A SPOTTER

I consider the use of a spotter crucial to intense training. A spotter lets you use advanced training techniques, monitors your form, and helps you break previous barriers. Not everyone is an effective spotter, however. There is a real art to spotting. Here are some guidelines for selecting a good spotter:

• The spotter must have the mental capacity to be as focused in the workout as you are.

• He/she is knowledgeable enough in physiology to immediately know if you're working the right muscles.

• He/she has the ability to prompt you on proper form and then correct you if necessary.

• He/she is a good communicator, capable of reading your nonverbal responses to workout exertion.

Remember, you may choose the best spotter in the world, but maximum intensity in every workout is still your responsibility.

THE INTENSITY SET

Before training a particular body part, perform what I call the intensity set. Select your basic exercise for the body part you're going to work. Then take an empty bar or the lightest weight possible. Complete each rep very slowly, keeping constant tension on the working muscles throughout the range of motion. Never relax, not even for an instant.

Once you contract the muscle, hold it as tightly as you can. Then pull it back to the starting position with the opposing muscle group. Make the exercise so intense that the muscle gives out after 10 reps. Put this same amount of concentration into every rep and every set you do.

ROUTINES

By incorporating pyramid sets, exhaustion sets, and fascial stretching, the following routines are designed to help you achieve the greatest increase in muscular size, definition, and strength. Novice bodybuilders should start with the beginning routine and eventually progress to the intermediate routine. How fast you advance is based on your state of nutrition and mental acuity. In other words, if you're following the nutrition program with 100 percent dedication and consistency, while remaining mentally focused in the gym, you should progress rather quickly to a higher level of training.

The six-day routine is written for advanced, well-nourished bodybuilders. Please realize that you will have to work up to this level of training—so consider this routine an example of what can be achieved. Please adjust your own reps, sets, and poundages to your individual training level and current muscular weight. Again, your training capabilities depend on your state of nutrition and training experience.

Unlike other muscles, the calves and abdominals can be worked on consecutive days. Remember to start each body part workout with an intensity set.

FOUR-DAY BEGINNING ROUTINE

Monday
Legs/Arms/Abs Exercise/Stretch	Pyramid Sets/Reps	Exhaustion Sets/Reps
Squats	3/10–6	1–2/15–25
Quad stretch		
Leg press	3/10–6	1–2/15–25
Quad stretch		
Leg curl	3/10–6	1–2/15–25
Forward hamstring stretch		
Seated calf raise		2/50–100
Calf squats		
Standing calf raise		2/25–50
Calf squats		
Dumbbell curls	3/10–6	1–2/15–25
Biceps stretch		
Spider curls	3/10–6	1–2/15–25
Biceps stretch		
Cable curls	3/10–6	1–2/15–25
Biceps stretch		
Lying triceps extension	3/10–6	1–2/15–25
Triceps stretch		
Triceps pressdown (strict)	3/10–6	1–2/15–25
Triceps stretch		
Triceps kickbacks	3/10–6	1–2/15–25
Triceps stretch		
Roman chair sit-ups	5/25–50	
Abdominal stretch		

Tuesday
Chest/Shoulders /Back/Calves Exercise/Stretch	Pyramid Sets/Reps	Exhaustion Sets/Reps
Bench press	3/10–6	1–2/15–25
Parrillo dips		
Incline dumbbell presses	3/10–6	1–2/15–25
Pec stretch		
Cable crossovers	3/10–6	1–2/15–25
Pec stretch		
Behind-the-neck presses	3/10–6	1–2/15–25
Shoulder stretch		
Seated dumbbell press	3/10–6	1–2/15–25
Delt stretch at dip bars		
Side lateral raises	3/10–6	1–2/15–25
Shoulder stretch		

Rich Gaspari goes for one more rep!
Photo by Jim Amentler.

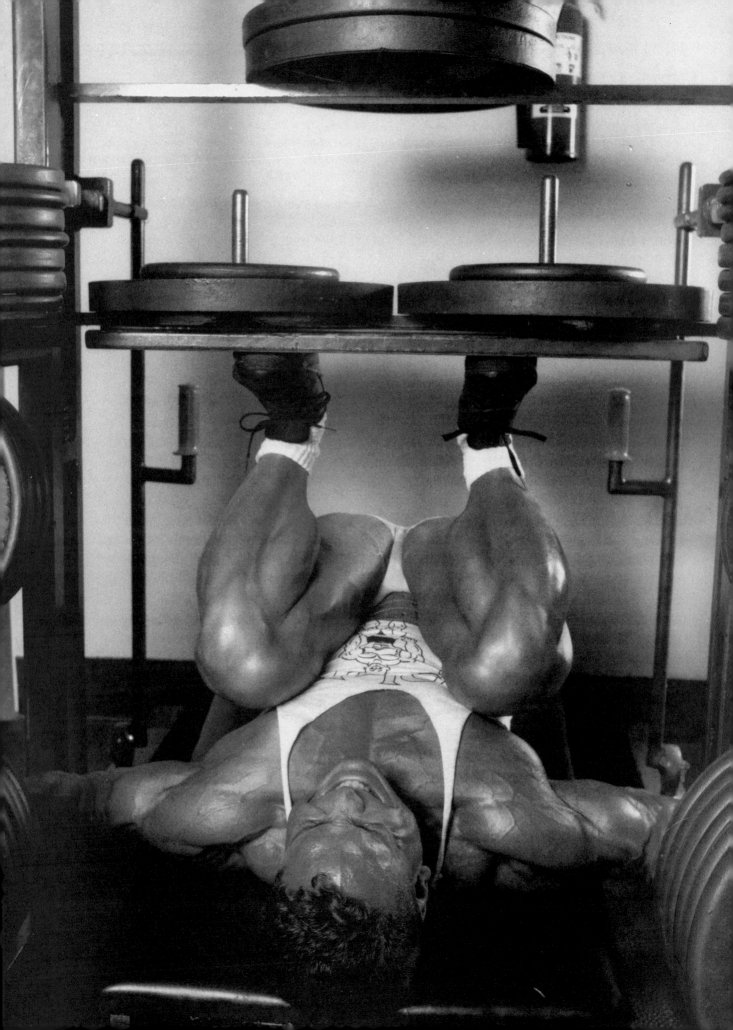

FOUR-DAY BEGINNING ROUTINE *(Continued)*

Tuesday
Chest/Shoulders
/Back/Calves

Exercise/Stretch	Pyramid Sets/Reps	Exhaustion Sets/Reps
T-bar rows	3/10–6	1–2/15–25
Lat stretch		
Wide-grip pulldowns	3/10–6	1–2/15–25
Lat stretch		
Close-grip pulldowns	3/10–6	1–2/15–25
Lat stretch		
Bent-over rows	3/10–6	1–2/15–25
Lat stretch		
Cable crunch	3/25	
Abdominal stretch		

Thursday
Legs/Arms/Abs

Exercise/Stretch	Pyramid Sets/Reps	Exhaustion Sets/Reps
Squats (narrow stance)	3/10–6	1–2/15–25
Hip stretch		
Leg press	3/10–6	1–2/15–25
Quad stretch		
Straight-leg deadlift	3/10–6	1–2/15–25
Butterfly		
Seated calf raise	3/15–25	2/50–100
Calf stretch		
Standing calf raise	3/15–25	2/25–50
Calf stretch		
Peak curls	3/10–6	1–2/15–25
Biceps stretch		
Preacher curls	3/10–6	1–2/15–25
Biceps stretch		
Cable curls	3/10–6	1–2/15–25
Biceps stretch		
Skull crushers	3/10–6	1–2/15–25
Triceps stretch		
Triceps pressdown (strict)	3/10–6	1–2/15–25
Triceps stretch		
Triceps kickbacks	3/10–6	1–2/15–25
Triceps stretch		
Roman chair sit-ups	5/25–50	

Abdominal
stretch

Friday
Chest/Shoulders
/Back/Abs

Exercise/Stretch	Pyramid Sets/Reps	Exhaustion Sets/Reps
Incline bench press	3/10–6	1–2/15–25
Pec stretch		
Dumbbell presses	3/10–6	1–2/15–25
Parrillo dips		
Cable crossovers	3/10–6	1–2/15–25
Pec stretch		
Behind-the-neck presses	3/10–6	1–2/15–25
Shoulder stretch		
Side lateral raises	3/10–6	1–2/15–25
Delt stretch at bar		
Wide-grip pulldowns	3/10–6	1–2/15–25
Lat stretch		
Close-grip pulldowns	3/10–6	1–2/15–25
Lat stretch		
Bent-over rows	3/10–6	1–2/15–25
Lat stretch		
Cable crunch	5/25–50	
Abdominal stretch		

FIVE-DAY INTERMEDIATE ROUTINE

Monday
Chest/Shoulders
/Arms/Abs

Exercise/Stretch	Pyramid Sets/Reps	Exhaustion Sets/Reps
Bench press	3/10–6	1–2/15–25
Pec stretch		
Incline bench press	3/10–6	1–2/15–25
Parrillo dips		

In my gym, we have a special cable crossover machine with adjustable pulleys so that you can work your pecs from different angles, as Bob Cicherillo demonstrates.
Photo by Jimmie D. King.

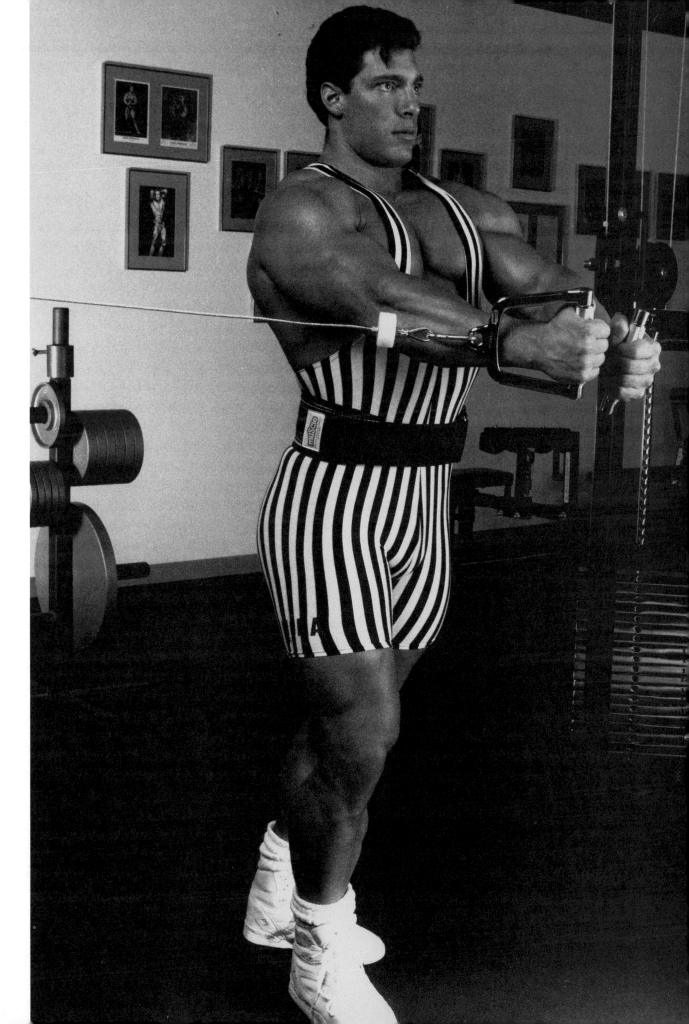

FIVE-DAY INTERMEDIATE ROUTINE *(Continued)*

Monday Chest/Shoulders /Arms/Abs Exercise/Stretch	Pyramid Sets/Reps	Exhaustion Sets/Reps
Bench-to-the- neck press Pec stretch	3/10–6	1–2/15–25
Behind-the-neck- press Narrow-grip skin-the-cat	3/10–6	1–2/15–25
Shoulder wrist rows Narrow-grip skin-the-cat	3/10–6	1–2/15–25
Lying triceps extension Triceps stretch	3/10–6	1–2/15–25
Triceps pressdown (cheat method) Triceps stretch	3/10–6	1–2/15–25
Dumbbell curls Biceps stretch	3/10–6	1–2/15–25
Preacher curls Biceps stretch	3/10–6	1–2/15–25

Tuesday Legs/Calves/ Traps/Abs Exercise/Stretch	Pyramid Sets/Reps	Exhaustion Sets/Reps
Deadlift Inner thigh/ hamstring stretch	3/10–6	1–2/15–25
Leg press Hip stretch	3/10–6	1–2/15–25
Seated calf raise Calf squat		1–2/50–100
Standing calf raise Calf squat		1–2/25–50
Shrugs Delt stretch at bar	3/10–6	1–2/15–25
Roman chair sit-ups (weighted)	4/25–50	

Abdominal stretch		
Cable crunch Abdominal stretch	3/25–50	

Thursday Back/Arms/ Legs/Calves/Abs Exercise/Stretch	Pyramid Sets/Reps	Exhaustion Sets/Reps
T-bar rows Lat stretch	3/10–6	1–2/15–25
Wide grip pulldowns to the back Lat stretch	3/10–6	1–2/15–25
Close grip pulldowns to the front Twisting stretch	3/10–6	1–2/15–25
Bent-over rows Twisting stretch	3/10–6	1–2/15–25
Peak curls Biceps stretch	3/10–6	1–2/15–25
Preacher curls Biceps stretch	3/10–6	1–2/15–25
Leg extensions Quad stretch	3/10–6	1–2/15–25
Leg curl Forward hamstring stretch	3/10–6	1–2/15–25
Seated calf raise Calf stretch		1–2/50–100
Standing calf raise Calf stretch		1–2/25–50
Roman chair sit-ups (weighted) Abdominal stretch	5/25–50	

Friday Chest/Triceps/ Shoulders Exercise/Stretch	Pyramid Sets/Reps	Exhaustion Sets/Reps
Bench press Parrillo dips	3/10–6	1–2/15–25
Decline bench press	3/10–6	1–2/15–25

Exercise/Stretch	Pyramid Sets/Reps	Exhaustion Sets/Reps
Medium-grip skin-the-cat		
Incline cable flyes	3/10–6	1–2/15–25
Medium-grip skin-the-cat		
Skullcrushers	3/10–6	1–2/15–25
Triceps stretch		
Triceps pressdown	3/10–6	1–2/15–25
Triceps stretch		
Shoulder wrist rows	3/10–6	1–2/15–25
Shoulder rhomboid stretch		
Side lateral raises	3/10–6	1–2/15–25
Shoulder rhomboid stretch		

Saturday
Legs/Calves/Back/Abs

Exercise/Stretch	Pyramid Sets/Reps	Exhaustion Sets/Reps
Squats	3/10–6	1–2/15–25
Quad stretch		
Stiff-leg deadlift	3/10–6	1–2/15–25
Forward hamstring stretch		
Seated calf raise		1–2/50–100
Calf squat		
Standing calf raise		1–2/25–50
Calf squat		
Seated rows	3/10–6	1–2/15–25
Lat stretch		
Wide-grip pulldowns	3/10–6	1–2/15–25
Lat stretch		
Close-grip pulldowns	3/10–6	1–2/15–25
Lat stretch		
Cable crunches	4/25–50	
Abdominal stretch		

SIX-DAY ADVANCED ROUTINE

Monday
Chest/Back/Abs

Exercise/Stretch	Pyramid Sets/Reps	Exhaustion Sets/Reps
Bench press	3/10–6	1–2/15–25
Medium-grip skin-the-cat		
Decline bench press	3/10–6	1–2/15–25
Parrillo dips		
Incline dumbbell press	3/10–6	1–2/15–25
Medium-grip skin-the-cat		
Cable crossovers	3/15–25	1–2/15–25
Pec stretch		
Standing calf raises		1–2/25–50
Calf stretch		
T-bar rows	3/10–6	1–2/15–25
Lat stretch		
Seated rows	3/10–6	1–2/15–25
Lat stretch		
Wide grip pulldowns to the back	3/10–6	1–2/15–25
Lat stretch		
Close grip pulldowns to the front	3/10–6	1–2/15–25
Lat stretch		
Bent-over rows	3/10–6	1–2/15–25
Lat stretch		
Roman chair sit-ups	3/25–50	
Abdominal stretch		
Leg lifts	3/25	

Tuesday
Shoulders/Arms/Abs/Calves

Exercise/Stretch	Pyramid Sets/Reps	Exhaustion Sets/Reps
Behind-the-neck press	3/10–6	1–2/15–25
Shoulder stretch		
Front lateral raises	3/10–6	1–2/15–25

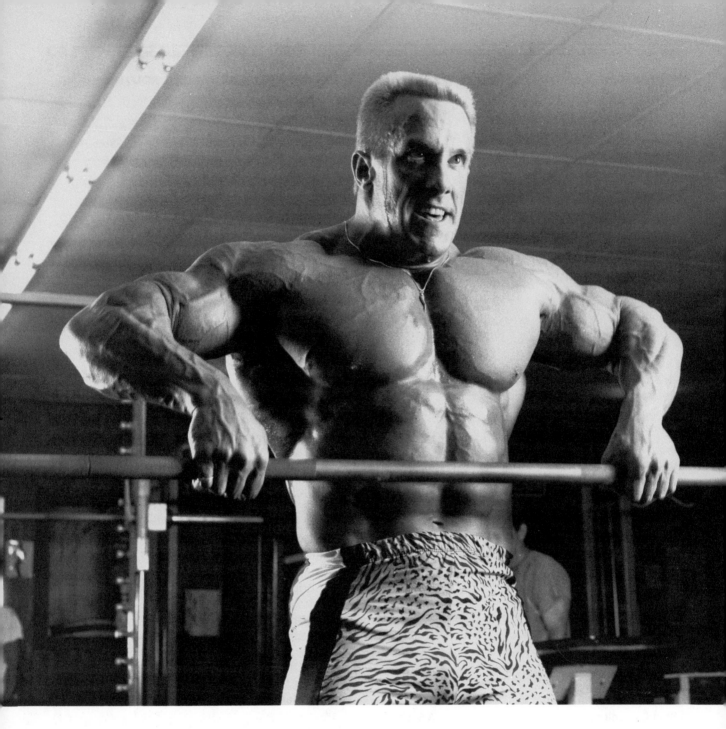

Intensity has a face: Dean Caputo! Photo by J. M. Manion.

SIX-DAY ADVANCED ROUTINE (Continued)

Tuesday Shoulders/Arms /Abs/Calves Exercise/Stretch	Pyramid Sets/Reps	Exhaustion Sets/Reps
Narrow-grip skin-the-cat		
Side lateral raises	3/10–6	1–2/15–25
Delt stretch at dip bars		
Bent-over lateral raises	3/10–6	1–2/15–25
Delt stretch at dip bars		
Dumbbell curls Biceps stretch	3/10–6	1–2/15–25
Preacher curls Biceps stretch	3/10–6	1–2/15–25

Exercise/Stretch	Pyramid Sets/Reps	Exhaustion Sets/Reps
Spider curls	3/10–6	1–2/15–25
Biceps stretch		
Lying triceps extensions	3/10–6	1–2/15–25
Triceps stretch		
Triceps pushdowns	3/10–6	1–2/15–25
Triceps stretch		
Skullcrushers	3/10–6	1–2/15–25
Triceps stretch		
Triceps kickbacks	3/10–6	1–2/15–25
Triceps stretch		
Cable crunches	3/25–50	
Seated calf raises		1–2/50–100

Wednesday
Legs/Calves/Abs

Exercise/Stretch	Pyramid Sets/Reps	Exhaustion Sets/Reps
Squats/wide stance	3/10–6	1–2/15–25
Hip stretch		
Leg press	3/10–6	1–2/15–25
Hip stretch		
Leg extensions	3/10–6	1–2/15–25
Quad stretch		
T-bar hamstring lift	3/10–6	1–2/15–25
Forward hamstring stretch		
Standing calf raises		1–2/25–50
Calf stretch		
Roman chair sit-ups	3/25	
Hanging leg raise	3/25	
Abdominal stretch		

Thursday
Legs/Back/Abs/ Calves

Exercise/Stretch	Pyramid Sets/Reps	Exhaustion Sets/Reps
Incline bench press	3/10–6	1–2/15–25
Medium-grip skin-the-cat		
Dumbbell bench press	3/10–6	1–2/15–25

Exercise/Stretch	Pyramid Sets/Reps	Exhaustion Sets/Reps
Parrillo dips		
Incline cable flyes	3/10–6	1–2/15–25
Pec stretch		
Cable crossovers	3/15–25	1–2/15–25
Pec stretch		
Wide-grip pullups	3/10–6	1–2/15–25
Lat stretch		
Close-grip pullups	3/10–6	1–2/15–25
Lat stretch		
Seated rows	3/10–6	1–2/15–25
Lat stretch		
T-bar rows	3/10–6	1–2/15–25
Lat stretch		
Bent-over dumbbell rows	3/10–6	1–2/15–25
Lat stretch		
Cable crunches	3/10–6	1–2/15–25
Abdominal stretch		
Standing calf raise		1–2/25–50
Calf squat		

Friday
Shoulders/Arms /Abs/Calves

Exercise/Stretch	Pyramid Sets/Reps	Exhaustion Sets/Reps
Seated dumbbell press	3/10–6	1–2/15–25
Shoulder stretch		
Seated wrist rows	3/10–6	1–2/15–25
Shoulder stretch		
Front lateral raise	3/10–6	1–2/15–25
Delt stretch at dip bars		
Side cable lateral raise	3/10–6	1–2/15–25
Delt stretch at dip bars		
Peak curls	3/10–6	1–2/15–25
Wide-grip skin-the-cat		
Seated dumbbell curls	3/10–6	1–2/15–25

SIX-DAY ADVANCED ROUTINE *(Continued)*

Friday
Shoulders/Arms
/Abs/Calves

Exercise/Stretch	*Pyramid Sets/Reps*	*Exhaustion Sets/Reps*
Wide-grip skin-the-cat		
Spider curls	3/10–6	1–2/15–25
Triceps stretch		
Lying triceps extension	3/10–6	1–2/15–25
Triceps stretch		
Triceps kickbacks	3/10–6	1–2/15–25
Triceps stretch		
Roman chair sit-ups	3/25	
Abdominal stretch		
Hanging leg raise	3/25	
Seated calf raises		1–2/50–100
Calf stretch		

Saturday
Legs/Calves/Abs

Exercise/Stretch	*Pyramid Sets/Reps*	*Exhaustion Sets/Reps*
Squats (narrow stance)	3/10–6	1–2/15–25
Quad stretch		
Leg press	3/10–6	1–2/15–25
Quad stretch		
Deadlift	3/10–6	1–2/15–25
Butterfly		
Leg curl	3/10–6	1–2/15–25
Inner thigh/ hamstring stretch		
Seated calf raise		1–2/50–100
Calf squat		
Standing calf raise		1–2/25–50
Calf squat		
Cable Crunch	3/25	
Abdominal Stretch		

ADVANCED TECHNIQUES

As you progress in your training, consider using advanced techniques in your routines. These techniques take you to a new level of intensity—but only if you put every ounce of effort into them and take in enough calories and nutrients for proper recovery.

FORCED REPS

Forced reps let you train past failure. After your last heavy set on an exercise, have your spotter lift the weight just past your sticking point. Then take over from there. Forced reps work the muscle very hard. I like to see bodybuilders pyramid up to a one-rep maximum and afterward do several forced reps. That's muscular overload at its best!

NEGATIVES

Negatives, in which just the eccentric or lowering portion of the exercise is performed, enhance neuromuscular efficiency—the ability to recruit a greater number of muscle fibers during muscular contraction.

Negatives build a quick-firing muscle, and you become stronger as a result. In addition, spotted, heavy negatives will increase your golgi tendon reflex threshold.

Your muscles can lower more weight than they can raise. So even though you've pushed the muscles to the max on your heavy pyramid sets, you can continue to do more work with negative reps. I suggest that you do some negatives after your heaviest set.

SUPERSETS

An excellent intensity builder, a superset is a pair of exercises performed one after the other without rest in between. You can superset exercises for opposing muscles, such as biceps and triceps, or exercises that work the same muscle, such as leg presses and leg extensions.

PUSH-PULL

As an intensity technique, push-pull has two different meanings in bodybuilding. The first is simply a method of supersetting in which you alternate pushing exercises such as behind-the-neck presses with pulling exercises such as upright rows.

Push-pull also refers to a type of split routine in which muscles that involve pushing are trained on separate days from those muscles that involve pulling. For example, on one day you'd work your chest and triceps; on the next day, your back and biceps. Push-pull routines are excellent for increasing strength levels.

REVERSE-EXHAUSTION

This technique involves working a muscle group first with a multijoint or compound movement such as a bench press or bent-over row, then following it with a single-joint or isolation exercise such as dumbbell rows. The opposite of this technique is pre-exhaustion, which involves supersetting an isolation exercise with a multijoint movement.

BELIEVE IN YOURSELF

As you train hard, believe in your ability to push yourself to the max. If you don't believe you can get the best workout of your life, you won't. But if you believe in yourself, you will.

I once worked with a bodybuilder who had never weighed more than 237. After competing in the Junior Nationals, he plotted a goal to go from 199 to 300 pounds. Each week, he gained three pounds. He got all the way up to 270 until someone told him he couldn't make it to 300 pounds. Sadly, he never gained a pound after that. He stopped believing in himself. Don't fall into this mental trap. When your attitude changes, everything changes. When you know you can do it, you can.

NUTRITION AND ADVANCED TRAINING

The more advanced your training becomes, the more attention you must pay to nutrition and supplementation. A great physique is not built solely by working out harder or eating more. It is built by adhering to metabolism-building nutrition and by increasing your nutrient levels through the use of nutritional supplements. As you stress your physique and push toward your potential, you'll require greater levels of nutrients just to recover from your workouts and to build more muscle.

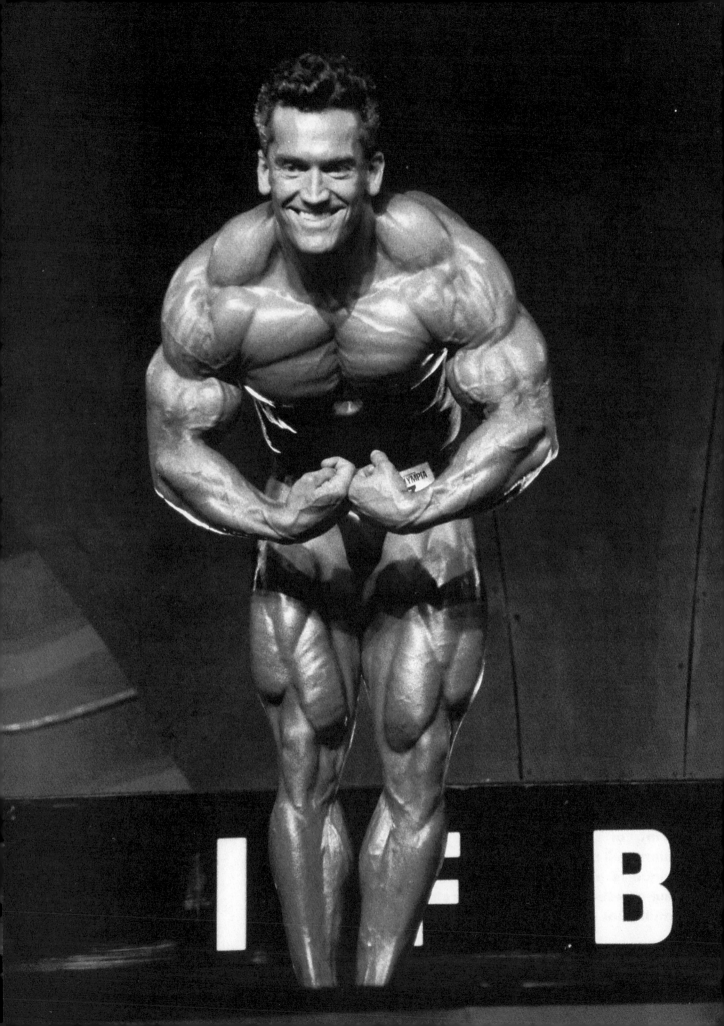

ELEVEN
CHARTING YOUR PROGRESS

As you continue to work toward your physique goals, you should monitor your progress along the way—so that you can continue to make gains.

Often, it is necessary to fine-tune your nutrition and training. You may have to eat more (or less) food, add more workouts to your routines, or increase or decrease your aerobics—all to achieve your objectives.

To make the right adjustments in your nutrition and training, you must analyze your body composition (the amount of body fat and muscle on your physique) on a weekly basis. Properly used and understood, body-composition testing lets you monitor your body from week to week, so that you can make the appropriate changes in your diet and training. It takes the guesswork out of how well your program is working and lets you see how much progress you're making. For example, if you gained two pounds last week, but those pounds were all fat, then you have not made any real progress.

Another essential component of my nutrition and training program is a system I developed for monitoring body composition. It's called BodyStat Charting. It uses skinfold calipers, the most accurate testing method for people below 15-percent body fat, and applies special calculations to give you an accurate assessment of your ratio of body weight to body fat, percentage of body fat, pounds of body fat, and pounds of muscle mass.

HOW IT WORKS

To use BodyStat Charting, you need a skinfold caliper device. This measures the thickness of a fold of skin with its underlying layer of fat. Skinfold calipers have springs that exert pressure on the skinfold and an accurate scale that measures the thickness in millimeters. Because of the locations of these skinfolds, you cannot measure yourself. Another person must take your measurements. This person should do it each time and measure in the same place each time.

If you're right-handed, take the calipers in your right hand. With your left hand, pull out the fold of skin with its underlying

Lee Labrada is known for his symmetry . . . but check out the muscle mass! Photo by J. M. Manion.

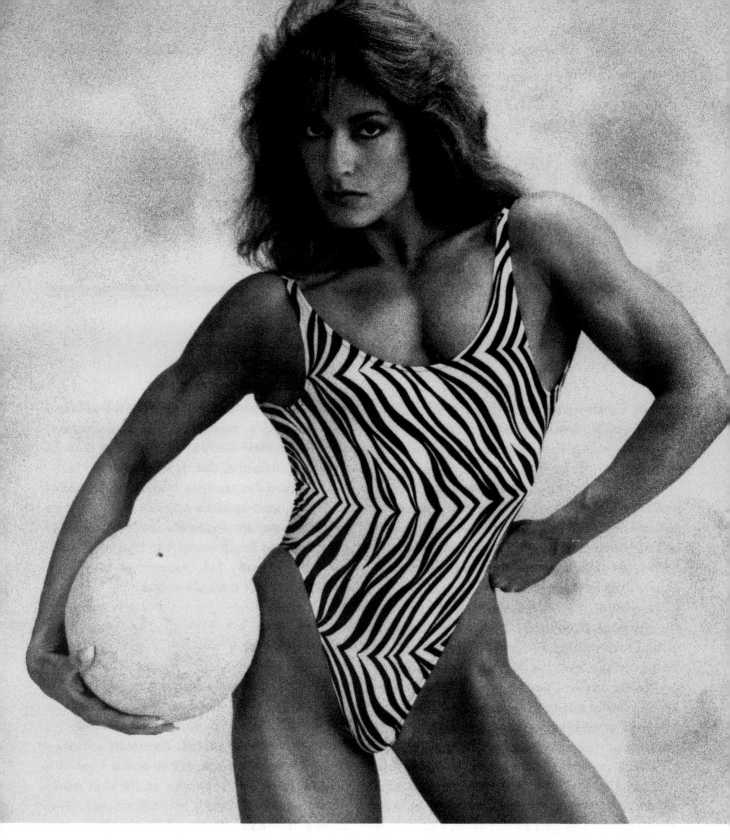

Patty Sanchez is a well known bodybuilder and a hard-working official with the International Federation of Bodybuilders (IFBB). Photo by Paul B. Goode.

layer of fat and grasp it between your thumb and forefinger. Don't worry about pinching muscle; it's so firm that it won't be taken up with the skin and body fat.

Place the jaws of the caliper on the skinfold. The jaws should be about ¼ inch from the fingers of your left hand. Completely release the trigger of the caliper so that the entire force of the jaws is on the skinfold. Don't release the fingers of your left hand while you take the readings.

The jaws will slide slightly to a lower reading as they are first applied. This happens because interstitial fluid is being squeezed from the skin. In seconds, the sliding will stop. At this point, the reading on the scale of the calipers should be read and recorded.

Skinfolds are measured at nine strategic locations on the body:

1. Pec. Measure about one inch below the collarbone and three to four inches out from the inside edge of the pectoral muscle. If you're measuring a woman, be sure to stay on the pec and avoid breast tissue. Pull the skinfold in a horizontal direction.

2. Subscapular. Locate the middle of the scapula (shoulder blade) and measure about one inch in toward the spine. Pull the skinfold in a vertical direction.

3. Biceps. Measure in the middle of the biceps muscle. Pull the skinfold in a vertical direction.

4. Triceps. Measure at the bottom of the inside triceps head. Pull the skinfold in a vertical direction.

5. Kidney. Locate the dimple or indentation above the gluteal muscles. Go up about two inches and out about two inches. Pull the skinfold in a horizontal direction.

6. Suprailiac. Measure about halfway between the navel and the top of the hipbone. This should be at or near the area where the obliques and abdominals meet. Pull the skinfold in a horizontal direction.

7. Abdominals. Measure about one inch to left of the navel or one inch to the right and one inch down. Pull the skinfold in a vertical direction.

8. Quadriceps. Measure in the middle of the quadriceps. If the area is too tight, move up one or two inches to get a reading. Pull the skinfold in a vertical direction.

9. Medial calf. Measure the middle of the inside head. If that area is too tight, move up one or two inches. Pull the skinfold in a vertical direction.

INTERPRETING THE NUMBERS

After recording the nine measurements, make the following calculations to determine your body composition:

1. Add the nine measurements and divide the total by your body weight. This figure gives you the ratio of body fat to body weight.

2. Multiply that ratio by .27 to get your percentage of body fat.

3. Multiply your percentage of body fat by your body weight to yield your pounds of body fat.

4. Subtract the pounds of body fat from your total body weight to calculate the pounds of lean mass.

Here's an example to illustrate how these calculations work:

1. After adding your nine BodyStat Charting measurements, you get a total of 65. Divide 65 by your body weight (200) to get a body fat to body weight ratio of .32.

2. Multiply your body weight to body fat ratio (.32) by .27 to get a body fat percentage of 8%.

3. Multiply your body weight (200) by your percentage of body fat (8%) to get 16 pounds of body fat.

4. Subtract the pounds of body fat (16) from your body weight (200) to get your total lean muscle mass of 184 pounds.

TAKING ACTION

You've taken the nine measurements and performed the four calculations to determine your body composition. Now you're ready to analyze the data and plan the appropriate course of action. Your plan depends on whether your principal concern is to lose body fat or to gain muscle mass.

MASS-BUILDING SOLUTIONS

When you're eating to gain muscle mass, several different changes can occur in your body composition. Here's what you should do in each case:

You're losing muscle. Clearly, you need to increase your intake of lean proteins, starchy carbohydrates, and fibrous carbohydrates. Add about 300 to 500 calories each day until your body-composition readings indicate a gain in muscle mass. Additionally, train with heavier weights and incorporate advanced techniques into your routines.

You're gaining muscle and maintaining body fat. This is an ideal state for mass-building. You'll need to increase your calories to support the additional muscular gain.

You're gaining muscle and losing body fat. As long as your body-fat and energy levels don't drop too much, you're in an optimum state.

You're gaining muscle and body fat. You should be gaining weight at the rate of one pound a week per 100 pounds of body weight. Gaining faster that than could lead to increased body fat. Where levels of body fat are concerned, men, on the average, should go no higher than 12 percent body fat; and women, no higher than 18 percent. As long as your body fat stays within these suggested levels, you're fine. If not, you may need to make a few changes. Review your nutrition program to make sure that you're eating the right foods in the proper combinations. If body-fat levels exceed the suggested limits, cut back on your calories and/or increase your aerobics as well as the intensity of your workouts.

You're maintaining muscle and gaining body fat. Your body may be entering a fat-producing phase. That being the case, you need to boost your metabolism. Stay stricter with your nutrition, increase your aerobics, and up the intensity of your workouts. Concentrate on losing about a half pound of body fat a week until this trend reverses itself. Also, increase your aerobics to as much as twice a day.

You're maintaining muscle and body fat. You've hit a plateau. Increase your caloric intake for a few weeks to see if you can start gaining muscle again. To shock your body into new growth, adjust your workouts. Lift heavier weights, change exer-

Tonya Knight trains for cuts and mass. Photo by Jim Amentler.

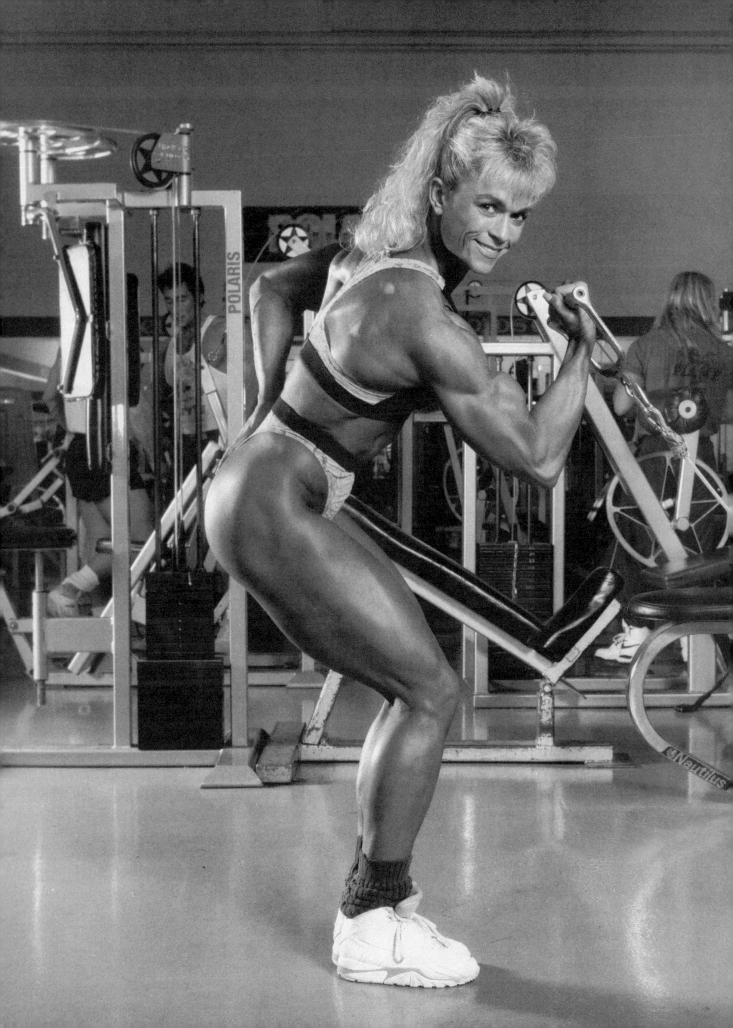

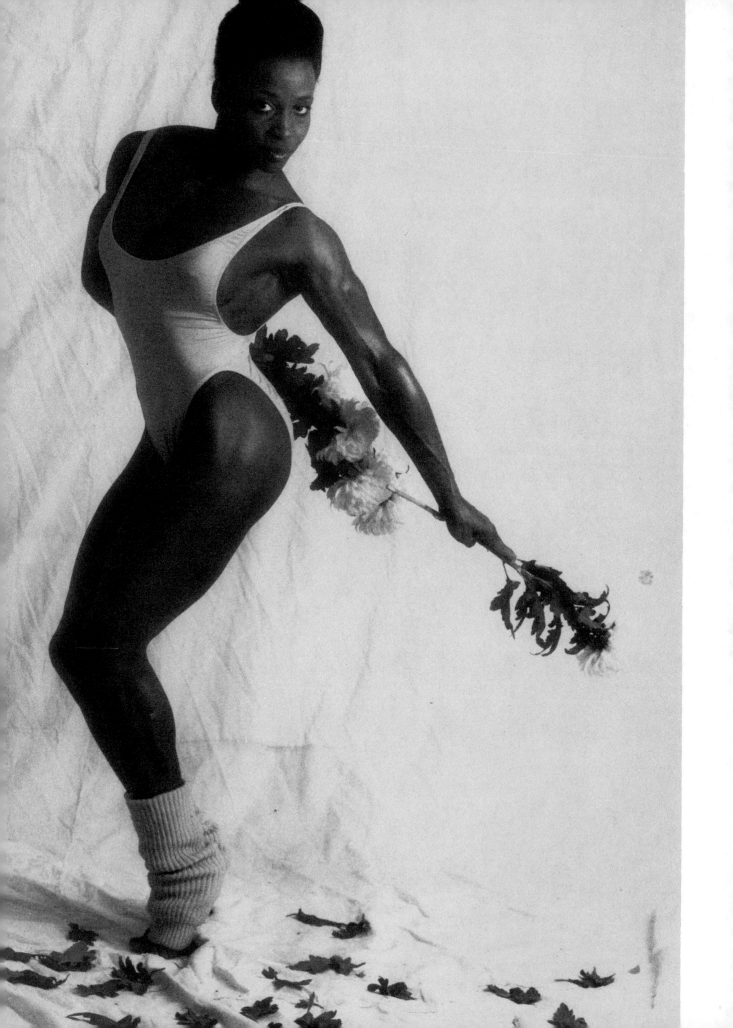

cises, or adopt a new routine. To help lose body fat, increase your aerobics.

You're maintaining lean mass and losing body fat. Although this is a desirable balance to be for losing body fat, your body can't create muscle in this state. You should, therefore, increase your caloric intake by 300 to 500 calories every several days until you gain at the rate of one pound a week per 100 pounds of body weight.

FAT-FIGHTING SOLUTIONS

You should try to lose body fat at the rate of one pound a week. If you lose faster than that, some of the loss may be muscle. While you attempt to lose body fat, an analysis of your body composition can reveal a number of different outcomes. Here's what you should do in each case:

You're losing body fat and maintaining muscle. Everything is working. Your nutrition, supplementation, and training are producing the desired effect. Don't change a thing.

You're maintaining body fat and muscle. You've hit a plateau. Reduce your intake of starchy carbohydrates while increasing the duration, frequency, and intensity of your aerobics.

You're gaining body fat and maintaining muscle. Further restrict your intake of starchy carbohydrates. Increase the duration, frequency, and intensity of your aerobics.

You're losing body fat and muscle. Your metabolism may be slowing down. This means that you should increase your caloric intake to recharge your metabolism. Don't be afraid to eat more.

You're gaining or maintaining body fat while losing muscle. This is a critical state. Your metabolism is sluggish, and your body has begun to hoard fat and break down the protein in muscles for energy. To recharge your metabolism, increase your caloric intake for several days. Eat enough to gain a pound a week per 100 pounds of body weight. Then recheck your body composition in a few days. If you're still losing mass, increase your calories even more. In addition, train with heavy weights to build and maintain muscularity and eliminate high-repetition training, which could lead to a loss of muscle mass.

IT'S UP TO YOU

Many components of proper nutrition and training have been covered here. It's important to emphasize that these components do not work alone but rather in combination with each other. You must consistently follow all the components of these programs—not just one or two.

So now it's up to you. You have the nutrition and training information to get results. Add to that dedication, consistency, and commitment, and you have the power to create the ultimate physique.

Carla Dunlap has been a top bodybuilding pro for more than a decade. Photo by Paul B. Goode.

Appendix A: Questions and Answers

Q: I'm ready to start your nutrition program. I'd like to lose body fat right away and then put on weight later. Is this the right approach?

A: No! Regardless of how much fat you want to lose, start the diet with the goal of gaining a pound of week per 100 pounds of body weight at first. That way you can increase your muscle, which in turn boosts your metabolism so you can burn fat much faster. To do that, gradually increase your calories until you gain weight at the suggested rate.

Look at it this way: If you gain a pound a week for five weeks and lose a pound a week for five weeks, you'll gain more mass and be much leaner than if you tried to lose first and gain later. So try to put on weight for several weeks. You will be amazed at how much bigger—and leaner—you will get.

Q: I've been bodybuilding for about six years. I follow a strict diet of fish, chicken, vegetables, oatmeal, brown rice, and so forth, and I try to eat as much as you suggest. But I have trouble getting in more than 3,500 calories a day. I work out very intensely on a four-on, one-off program. My problem is that it's difficult for me to add muscle to my frame. What should I do?

A: You may think you cannot gain any more muscle, but, believe me, you can. Nutrition is the key. Most bodybuilders who fail to make gains simply do not eat enough. To increase your caloric intake to the necessary level, you have to train your body to process more nutrients. This is done by gradually increasing your calories.

When I tell women to work up to 6,000 calories a day and men up to 10,000 calories a day, I do not expect all those calories to come from food. I expect them to rely on caloric-dense supplements such as MCFA oil, carbohydrate supplements, and protein powders or bars.

Q: I've heard that you don't believe in the concept of overtraining. Could you clarify what you mean?

A: Overtraining is simply "underrecovery"—not taking in enough nutrients to fully recover from your workouts. If ample nutrients are not provided, killer workouts won't do any good. But once you get in the habit of making your nutrition as intense as your training, your workouts will be much more productive, and you'll see results in no time.

Q: In the off-season, I can't seem to gain any muscle. I feel as though I've reached a plateau, what should I do?

A: Many bodybuilders use the off-season to go off their diets, eating everything in sight and paying very little attention to mass-building nutrition. For competitive bodybuilders, the off-season is the time to put on muscle. To do that, you have to eat enough to increase your body weight. Even though it's the off-season, you must still stay strict on your diet. Eat the right foods (lean protein, starchy carbohydrates, and fibrous carbohydrates) in the right combinations and in multiple meals (five or six a day). In addition, use MCFA oil, a carbohydrate supplement, and a protein powder or bar to increase your daily caloric intake.

If you have reached a plateau, you are probably not doing any—or enough—off-season aerobics. Aerobics build your capillary beds for greater cardiovascular density, which means better oxygen and nutrient delivery to muscle tissue for growth. The better your cardiovascular density, the greater potential you have for building bigger muscles. Be consistent with aerobics in the off-season, follow a strict, nutritious diet, take your supplements, and you'll surpass that plateau in no time at all.

Q: I've heard that a person can digest only 30 grams of protein a meal. You recommend much more than that. Is all that protein really used or just washed out of the system? And, why do you recommend eating so much protein on a bodybuilding diet?

A: Hard-training bodybuilders need more protein than most individuals. The main reason is that intense training causes greater usage of amino acids by the muscles.

In working with top bodybuilders for 20 years, I have found that an intake of between 1.25 and 1.5 grams of protein a day per pound of body weight, along with adequate calories, supports muscular growth, repair, and recovery. As you train your metabolism to be more efficient—that is, to process more nutrients—you'll be able to digest, absorb, and utilize more protein. Stay aware of the effect of your diet on your gains. If you are making consistent progress, then you are eating the right amount of protein and other nutrients to support those gains. If your muscles in their flexed state ever feel soft, then your diet is probably deficient in protein and/or calories.

Q: If MCFAs are a triglyceride, will the supplement affect my cholesterol levels?

A: With its shorter chain structure, MCFA oil is utilized very differently from the harmful long-chain triglycerides found in fatty foods. It is burned up so rapidly in the body that very little is retained. In fact, research has shown that MCFAs do not increase overall cholesterol levels.

Q: How should I account for MCFA oil when I calculate my daily intake of calories and grams of protein, fat, and carbohydrate?

A: You need only account for the supplement's caloric content, which is 114 calories per tablespoon.

Q: Will I experience any side effects from taking MCFA oil?

A: Because it is a natural supplement, MCFA oil won't harm your body. It can, however, cause your body to undergo some changes. Although most people do not have any problems when they introduce it gradually into the diet, you may experience slight cramping and diarrhea when you begin taking the supplement. This is caused by the rapid digestion of the supplement. Decrease your usage of the supplement until your tolerance improves.

Q: I attended one of your seminars last year and heard you talk about the importance of fascial stretching. How do I incorporate stretching into my workout?

A: Fascial stretching should be a part of every workout. Do a few light stretches before training. I emphasize "light" here because overstretching cold muscles can promote injuries.

Then, stretch between every exercise set to stimulate muscular growth, enhance muscular shape and separation, and build strength. Other benefits include decreased muscle soreness, fewer injuries, and increased flexibility. Be sure to learn a variety of fascial stretching exercises for each muscle group by following the instructions in this book.

Q: I'm satisfied with my upper-body development, but my quadriceps and hamstrings seem to be lagging behind. Also, when I diet for a contest, my legs never get as cut as the rest of my body. What can I do to improve my legs in terms of both size and cuts?

A: First, let me address the issue of size. Whether you are trying to build your legs, arms, or any other muscle group, the most important thing is to consume plenty of quality calories from lean proteins, starchy carbohydrates, and fibrous carbohydrates. You can't expect to grow unless you gain weight. When it comes to leg training, keep two things in mind: form and intensity. You must use strict form throughout a complete range of motion, feel the muscle groups you're working, and give every set all-out effort. If you need more size on your legs, try pyramiding up to triples (3 repetitions a set) on regular squats and belt squats. Then finish with sets of 15 to 25 repetitions of shaping exercises,

such as leg extensions and curls, for cardiovascular density. Eliminate the heavy sets about one week before your competition. Use fascial stretching between every exercise set to bring out muscular size, separation, and shape.

To get your legs cut for a contest, you may need to increase your aerobics. Try 30 minutes to an hour of outdoor aerobics (running or cycling) every morning before breakfast and again after your last meal.

Q: After about two years of weight training, I don't seem to be getting the same results from workouts. How many sets and repetitions should I do, and do I need to use heavy poundages to keep growing?

A: It sounds as if your body has reached a new peak and now requires additional nutrients and more intense training. First of all, if you have stopped growing, it may be because of your diet. No matter how hard you train, you won't grow unless you eat properly and increase your calories. You should weigh all your food to make sure you are getting enough calories and the proper amounts of protein, carbohydrate, and fat. Concentrate on gaining weight at the rate of a pound a week per 100 pounds of body weight. As far as workouts are concerned, a combination of low repetitions/heavy poundages for muscle mass and high repetitions/lighter poundages for cardiovascular density is best. As you perform your workout, maintain a high level of intensity, especially during the last few repetitions of each set. Always concentrate on feeling the muscle group you are working, and have your training partner or a competent spotter help you with some forced repetitions. Be sure to use fascial stretching between every exercise set.

Q: During pre-contest training, how should I work out?

A: During contest preparation, many body-builders shift to lighter weights, thinking that this practice will sharpen muscularity. This is a big mistake, however. You should continue your heavy training to support the mass and density you have achieved up to this point. Reducing your poundages will only make you look softer and smaller.

By promoting further gains in muscle mass, heavy work during pre-contest training keeps your metabolism revved up. Remember, the more muscle you have, the faster your metabolism is for fat-burning and muscle-building.

In the final weeks before your competition, perform one or two additional high-rep sets at the end of each body-part workout in order to build cardiovascular density. By continuing your heavy work and combining it with high-rep sets, you can better achieve your contest peak.

Appendix B: Recipes

Healthy, low-fat foods do not have to taste boring or bland, especially if you use MCFA oil, spices, and other nutritious condiments in your food preparation. In this section, you'll find some delicious recipes for everything, from entrées to desserts. Use them as part of your nutrition program.

COOKING WITH MCFA OIL

MCFA oil is used in all of these recipes. Because it burns at 350 degrees, keep your heat no higher than 325 degrees when cooking. If the oil smokes, reduce heat quickly.

OATMEAL FLOUR

Oatmeal flour is used in many of these recipes. If you can't purchase this type of flour, you can easily make it. Place rolled oats in your food processor or blender and blend until the oatmeal becomes a very fine powder. Make oatmeal flour in quantity and store it in an airtight container.

POPCORN SALT

Popcorn salt has approximately 200–250 mg. of sodium per large pinch between your fingers. Always add your salt this way, without sprinkling directly from the container to avoid excessive salting of foods.

BREAKFAST FOODS

Barley Cakes

7 (200 g.) egg whites
½ cup barley flour
½ tsp. cinnamon
½ cup (100 g.) grated carrots
1 tbsp. MCFA oil

Beat egg whites. Combine other ingredients, and stir into egg whites. Cook in a moderately hot skillet which has been lightly sprayed with a non-stick spray. Make the pancakes small.

Nutritional value of entire recipe: 438 calories, 28.9 g. protein, 2.8 g. fat, 45 g. carbohydrate, 341 mg. sodium, and 714 g. potassium.

Variation: To make a dinner variation of barley cakes, substitute onion, zucchini, and garlic for the cinnamon. Barley cakes are best served with chicken. They keep well in plastic baggies to take with you to work or on the road.

Country Mexican Omelette

10 (300 g.) egg whites
1 cup (200 g.) boiled potatoes, sliced small and thin
4 oz. mild salsa
¼ cup (50 g.) sliced mushrooms
3 tbsp. MCFA oil

In a large bowl, coat potatoes with MCFA oil. Place potatoes and mushrooms in hot 12" nonstick skillet. Saute until mushrooms are tender. Pour egg whites on top of mixture and let cook until egg whites are almost done. Pour salsa on top and cover. Cook on low heat until completely done. Fold one side over. This omelette makes a hearty breakfast when served with oatmeal pancakes.

Nutritional value of entire recipe: 797 calories, 39.6 g. protein, .51 g. fat, 45.8 g. carbohydrate, 835.5 mg. sodium, and 1,439 g. potassium.

Crepes

1¼ cups (100 g.) oatmeal flour
7 (200 g.) egg whites
½ tsp. cinnamon
½ tsp. almond extract
2 tbsp. MCFA oil
½ cup water

Mix all ingredients into a batter and blend well. Because the batter should be somewhat thin, add more water as needed. In hot 8-inch skillet that has been lightly sprayed with a non-stick spray, pour just enough batter to cover the bottom of the skillet. Crepes should be very thin. Turn over when edges become easy to lift and cook at least one additional minute. Repeat process until batter is gone.

Nutritional value of entire recipe: 720 calories, 36 g. protein, 7.4 g. fat, 69.8 g. carbohydrate, 294 mg. sodium, and 630 g. potassium.

Oatmeal Pancakes

1¼ cups (100 g.) oatmeal flour
1 oz. powdered carbohydrate supplement
1½ tsp. cinnamon
¼ tsp. baking powder
¼ tsp. baking soda
2 tsp. pure vanilla
7 (200 g.) egg whites
1 tbsp. MCFA oil
⅓ cup water

Mix all dry ingredients in medium-sized bowl. Add rest of the ingredients and mix well with a wire whip. Heat griddle on medium heat until hot. Pour ⅛ cup of the batter onto griddle, turning when bubbles appear on the top. Cook for about 30 seconds and remove from griddle. Makes about 10–12 pancakes.

Nutritional value of entire recipe: 711 calories, 40 g. protein, 7.4 g. fat, 91.8 g. carbohydrate, 358 mg. sodium, and 802 g. potassium.

Turkey Sausage

½ tsp. fennel seeds
½ tsp. crushed red peppers
½ tsp. dried rosemary
14 oz. (400 g.) ground turkey
½ tsp. freshly ground black pepper
¼ tsp. salt substitute (optional)
4 tbsp. MCFA oil

Crush fennel, red pepper, and rosemary. Add turkey and all other ingredients. Mix well and form into eight patties. Cook over medium heat until lightly brown on both sides. Turkey sausage patties can be frozen for later use.

Nutritional value of entire recipe: 920 calories, 98.4 g. protein, 4.8 g. fat, 0 g. carbohydrate, 204 mg. sodium, and 1,280 g. potassium.

Turkey Sausage Gravy

2 tbsp. MCFA oil
¼ cup (20 g.) oatmeal flour
1 cup water

Take drippings from sausage and add oil. Cook in a small saucepan over medium heat. Stir in oatmeal flour. Slowly add water, stirring constantly until desired thickness. Add pepper and substitute salt to taste. This gravy is delicious served over biscuits.

Nutritional value of entire recipe: 306 calories, 2.8 g. protein, 1.5 g. fat, 13.6 g. carbohydrate, 0 mg. sodium, and 70.4 g. potassium.

MAIN DISHES

Chicken Fingers

1 medium (150 g.) chicken breast, partially frozen
1 tbsp. MCFA oil
¼ cup (20 g.) oatmeal
garlic
paprika
chili powder
pepper

Cut chicken into thin slices (1″ × ½″). Put in a bowl and toss with other ingredients, adding spices to taste. Place chicken strips on a cookie sheet that has been sprayed with non-stick spray. Bake at 400 degrees for 15 minutes.

Nutritional value of entire recipe: 387 calories, 38.7 g. protein, 4.8 g. fat, 17 g. carbohydrate, 75.5 mg. sodium, and 568 g. potassium.

Chicken Ratatouille

1 medium (300 g.) eggplant, peeled and sliced into ¼-inch slices
6 tbsp. MCFA oil
2 tbsp. oatmeal flour
garlic salt (to taste)
1 medium (80 g.) finely chopped onion
3 (450 g.) zucchini, washed and sliced
2 medium (300 g.) green peppers, seeded and diced
4 medium (700 g.) peeled and chopped tomatoes
4 (600 g.) chicken breasts, cooked and diced

Heat the oil on low heat in a large non-stick skillet. Add garlic salt and onion. Saute until tender but not brown. Toss the zucchini with 1 tbsp. flour and add to the skillet. Rinse and quarter eggplant slices, pat dry and dust with the remaining flour. Add to the skillet. Add green peppers, tomatoes, and cooked chicken. Cook uncovered until the vegetables are tender. Serve warm or cold. Makes 4 servings.

Nutritional value of entire recipe: 2134 calories, 162.2 g. protein, 14.5 g. fat, 162.8 g. carbohydrate, 329.5 mg. sodium, and 5,305 g. potassium.

Chicken Salad

4 boiled chicken breasts (600 g.), cooled and shredded
½ cup (100 g.) chopped lettuce
½ cup (100 g.) chopped celery
¼ cup (50 g.) minced onion
1 cup MCFA oil mayonnaise (See below in Sauces and Marinade section)
1 clove garlic minced or ½ tsp. garlic powder
¼ tsp. ginger
½ tsp. onion powder
pepper to taste

Place chicken and vegetables in medium bowl. In a smaller bowl, combine mayonnaise and spices. Mix well and pour over chicken and vegetables. Mix again. Scoop chicken salad onto tomato wedges.

Variation: Add 1 cup (200 g.) fresh or thawed frozen peas.

Nutritional value of entire recipe: 2,070 calories, 158. g. protein, 16.7 g. fat, 12.8 g. carbohydrate, 534 mg. sodium, and 2,761 g. potassium.

Fried Chicken

1¼ cups (100 g.) shredded wheat, finely crumbled up
¼ cup (21 g.) oat bran
1 tsp. onion powder
½ tsp. garlic powder
½ tsp. barbecue seasoning
½ tsp. coarse black pepper
1 tsp. Lemon and Herb Mrs. Dash
7 (1,000 g.) chicken breasts
5 tbsp. MCFA oil

Place chicken in medium-sized bowl and thoroughly coat with oil. Set aside. In another bowl, mix all other ingredients to form the breading. Dip chicken one piece at a time into the breading mixture and toss until coated thickly. Heat skillet with any remaining oil to 325 degrees. Place breaded chicken in heated skillet. Reduce heat and cover. Turn occasionally to cook evenly on all sides. Chicken is done when breading is all brown, and the meat is white, juicy, and tender. Be careful not to overcook, as this will dry out the chicken and make it tough.

Nutritional value of entire recipe: 2,191 calories, 257.4 g. protein, 22.7 g. fat, 95.9 g. carbohydrate, 503 mg. sodium, and 3,638 g. potassium.

Lemon Spiced Chicken

4 (600 g.) chicken breasts
8 tbsp. MCFA oil
4 tbsp. lemon juice
Lemon and Herb Mrs. Dash

Cut chicken into strips and place in medium-size bowl with oil and 1 tbsp. lemon juice. Coat chicken thoroughly. Place the chicken in a hot non-stick skillet and add other 3 tbsp. lemon juice. Sprinkle chicken with Mrs. Dash.

Cook over medium heat about 15 minutes or until chicken is done throughout.

Nutritional value of entire recipe: 1,640 calories, 140.9 g. protein, 11.6 g. fat, 8.6 g. carbohydrate, 301 mg. sodium, and 2,080 g. potassium.

Spiced Rice with Chicken

2 cups (200 g.) brown rice, soaked in water for 1 hour
3 (450 g.) chicken breasts
2 tsp. allspice
½ tsp. mace
3 tbsp. MCFA oil
½ to 1 tsp. pepper
½ tsp. No Salt (optional)

While rice is soaking, cut chicken into small pieces or grind it up in a food processor. Place chicken in a bowl with oil. Coat well. Place coated chicken in the same non-stick pan that you'll be cooking rice with. Sauté chicken with spices until chicken is done. Set aside. Drain rice and rinse well with cold water. Put 2 cups of water into the pan with chicken. Bring to a boil and add rice. Return to boil. Reduce heat, cover, and simmer until water is absorbed. Serves 4.

Nutritional value of entire recipe: 1,536 calories, 107 g. protein, 8.4 g. fat, 160.8 g. carbohydrate, 210 mg. sodium, and 1,464 g. potassium.

Turkey Chili

10½ oz. (300 g.) ground turkey
1 cup (200 g.) diced onion
2 cups (400 g.) kidney beans
3 tbsp. MCFA oil
½ cup (100 g.) chopped green pepper
2 14.5 oz cans (800 g.) whole peeled tomatoes, no sugar or salt added
3 tbsp. chili powder

On medium heat, sauté onion and turkey in oil until done, chopping turkey while stirring. Blend tomatoes. Add tomatoes, chili powder, beans, and green pepper to turkey and onion mixture. Simmer 30 to 40 minutes. Serves 4.

Nutritional value of entire recipe: 2,335 calories, 176.1 g. protein, 11.6 g. fat, 307.7 g. carbohydrate, 237 mg. sodium, and 6,946 g. potassium.

Vegetable Turkey Stew

¾ cup (150 g.) eggplant
¾ cup (150 g.) yellow squash
1 cup (200 g.) potato
1 cup (200 g.) cauliflower
¾ cup (150 g.) zucchini
1 cup (200 g.) onion
10-½ oz. (300 g.) ground turkey
3 tsp. garlic powder
2-14.4 oz. cans (800 g.) peeled whole tomatoes, no salt or sugar added
½ cup MCFA oil
⅓ cup MCFA oil

Chop up vegetables into bite-size chunks and place in a Dutch oven with ½ cup MCFA oil and 2 tsp. garlic powder. Cut turkey into bite-size chunks and place in non-stick skillet with ⅓ cup MCFA oil and 1 tsp. garlic powder. Sauté over low to medium heat until brown. Add turkey to vegetables and cook on top of stove for about five minutes, while stirring. Add blended tomatoes and simmer 30 to 40 minutes on low heat.

Nutritional value of entire recipe: 2,365 calories, 99.8 g. protein, 6.75 g. fat, 115.9 g. carbohydrate, 235 mg. sodium, and 5,341 g. potassium.

SIDE DISHES

Brown Rice and Lentils

5 cups water
1 cup (100 g.) brown rice
½ cup (100 g.) lentils
¼ cup (25 g.) chopped mushrooms
5 cloves garlic
2 tbsp. MCFA oil

Bring water to a hard boil and add rice. Reduce heat to a low boil. After 35 minutes, add lentils, mushrooms, and garlic. Turn heat down to simmer and let cook another 25 to 35 minutes or until all water is gone and lentils are soft. Stir occasionally to prevent sticking. Add MCFA oil to rice and lentils just before eating.

Nutritional value of entire recipe: 935 calories, 38.7 g. protein, 3 g. fat, 138.6 g. carbohydrate, 43 mg. sodium, and 1,107 g. potassium.

Hash Browns

4 medium (1,000 g.) potatoes
water
2 tbsp. finely chopped onion
½ tsp. garlic powder
2 tbsp. MCFA oil

Peel potatoes and cook in 1 inch boiling water for 30 minutes. Drain and cool, then grate and toss with onion, garlic powder, and pepper. Heat MCFA oil in a non-stick skillet on medium-low heat and place potato mixture in skillet, packing tightly and leaving a ¾-inch space around the edges. Cook over low heat for 12 minutes or until crust is formed. Cut into quarters and turn, then brown other side. Makes two servings.

Nutritional value of entire recipe: 1,000 calories, 21.45 g. protein, 1 g. fat, 173.6 g. carbohydrate, 33 mg. sodium, and 4,517 g. potassium.

Home Fries

2½ to 3 (600 g.) potatoes sliced in food processor or thinly sliced by hand
3 tbsp. MCFA oil
½ tsp. onion powder
½ tsp. garlic powder

dash of red pepper
¼ cup water

Place all ingredients except water in a large bowl and toss until potatoes are evenly coated with MCFA oil and spices. Place in a hot non-stick skillet, cover and let cook on medium heat for about 5 minutes. Pour water in skillet and turn potatoes with spatula. Cover again and let cook until potatoes are tender and lightly brown, stirring occasionally.

Nutritional value of entire recipe: 798 calories, 12.6 g. protein, .6 g. fat, 102.6 g. carbohydrate, 18 mg. sodium, and 2,447 g. potassium.

Lentil Delight

4 tbsp. MCFA oil
¼ cup (50 g.) dried onion
1 cup (200 g.) lentils, soaked overnight
¼ cup (50 g.) diced celery
¼ cup (50 g.) diced bell pepper

Place onions and MCFA oil over low heat in heavy pan. Stir one minute and add softened lentils, celery, and pepper. Cover tightly. Simmer until lentils are fully tender.

Nutritional value of entire recipe: 1,175 calories, 55.25 g. protein, 2.3 g. fat, 127.1 g. carbohydrate, 134.5 mg. sodium, and 1,946 g. potassium.

Green and Crunchy Salad

½ cup (100 g.) quartered Brussels sprouts
5 tbsp. MCFA oil
½ cup (100 g.) green beans, cut into ½ inch pieces
3 tbsp. lemon juice
½ cup (100 g.) chopped celery
2 tbsp. fresh or 1½ tsp. dried basil
¼ cup (50 g.) chopped bell pepper
2 tbsp. chopped parsley
2 tbsp. chopped green onion

Microwave sprouts and beans until tender but crunchy. Drain and chill. Chop remaining vegetables and combine them with sprouts and beans. Mix together ingredients for dressing. Shake well and pour over salad. Toss to coat vegetables and chill for one hour before eating.

Variation: Add ½ cup cooked rice.

Nutritional value of entire recipe: 660 calories, 5.8 g. protein, 4.7 g. fat, 20.9 g. carbohydrate, 150 mg. sodium, and 943 g. potassium.

SAUCES AND MARINADES

Barbecue Sauce

2 tbsp. MCFA oil
2 14½ oz. cans (400 g.) whole tomatoes
½ cup (100 g.) chopped onion
1 6-oz. can (200 g.) vegetable juice
2 cloves minced garlic

1 bay leaf
½ tsp. cloves
½ tsp. allspice
2 tsp. dry mustard
3 tbsp. vinegar
¼ cup (50 g.) celery stalk w/leaves
1 tsp. hot sauce
¼ cup (50 g.) chopped green pepper
2 tsp. natural hickory flavoring
3 pinches hickory smoke salt (optional)

In medium saucepan, sauté onion and garlic until tender in MCFA oil. Stir in remaining ingredients and bring to a boil. Reduce heat and simmer uncovered 30 minutes, stirring occasionally. Discard bay leaf and process sauce through a food mill or blender. Use barbecue sauce to baste or serve with chicken or turkey.

Cacciatore Sauce

2 tbsp. MCFA oil
¼ cup (50 g.) chopped green pepper
1 cup (200 g.) chopped onion
1 cup (200 g.) fresh chopped tomato
½ cup chopped parsley or ⅓ cup dried parsley
30 g. tomato paste (optional)
1 tsp. dried basil or 2 tbsp. fresh basil
1 tsp. dried oregano or 2 tbsp. fresh oregano

Place vegetables, MCFA oil, tomato paste, and herbs in medium saucepan or skillet. Mix well. Cover and simmer until vegetables are soft consistency, about 15 to 20 minutes. Cacciatore sauce is especially good over chicken or turkey, but try it over fish, zucchini, or eggs!

Creamy Tomato Dressing

6 tbsp. MCFA oil mayonnaise
6 tsp. lemon juice
½ tsp. dried onion
1 tsp. fresh basil
½ cup (100 g.) fresh chopped tomato

Blend on low speed in blender until creamy and thin enough to drizzle over salads or vegetables. Makes about ¾ cup. About 41 calories per tbsp.

Ginger Sauce for Vegetables

2 tbsp. MCFA oil
1 cup (200 g.) chopped onions
1 clove garlic, minced
1 tsp. grated fresh ginger or ½ tsp. dried ginger
2 tsp. lemon juice

Simmer onions and garlic in MCFA oil until soft. Stir in ginger and lemon juice. Simmer 5 minutes more to give flavors time to expand. Makes about ⅔ cup that can be refrigerated for later use.

Green Goddess Dressing

¾ cup MCFA oil mayonnaise
3 tbsp. snipped parsley
3 tbsp. chives or green onion
3 tbsp. dill leaves or 1½ tsp dried dillweed
1 tbsp. lemon juice
1 tbsp. MCFA oil

Mix ingredients, using additional lemon juice and MCFA oil to thin dressing as desired. Let sit a few minutes. Pour by spoonfuls over raw or cooked vegetables. Each tbsp. contains 83 calories.

Italian Marinade for Chicken or Fish

9 tbsp. MCFA oil
9 tbsp. lemon juice
1 tbsp. dried or 3 tbsp. fresh oregano
1 tsp. dried or 3 tbsp. fresh thyme
1 slice onion
1 garlic clove

Blend MCFA oil, lemon juice, and herbs with a fork. Add onion and garlic. Should be used for four to six chicken breasts. If you are cooking less chicken, use 2 to 3 tbsp. of the marinade and refrigerate leftover marinade. Marinate chicken or fish at least one hour before grilling.

MCFA Oil Mayonnaise

2 (70 g.) egg whites
2 tbsp. lemon juice
1 cup MCFA oil
1 tsp. dry mustard

Beat egg whites in blender on low speed. Add lemon juice and dry mustard. Continue to blend and slowly drizzle in MCFA oil. Continue blending until smooth. Keep refrigerated! Makes about 1½ cups mayonnaise. MCFA oil mayonnaise has 78 calories per tbsp.

Mexican Bean Dip

1 cup (200 g.) cooked pinto beans
¾ cup (150 g.) finely chopped tomato
4 tbsp. MCFA oil
½ tsp. chili powder
½ tsp. cumin

Puree beans in food processor or mash with fork. Add rest of ingredients and continue to blend.

Variation: Add 1 clove garlic, ½ cup minced onion, and some finely chopped chili pepper to taste. Substitute kidney beans for pinto beans.

Tartar Sauce for Fish

½ cup MCFA oil mayonnaise
1 to 2 tbsp. green onion or fresh chives
1 tsp. lemon juice
1 tsp. dried tarragon or 1 tbsp. fresh tarragon, scissor snipped
1 tsp. dried dill weed or 1 tbsp. fresh dillweed

Mix all ingredients with fork until well blended. Serve with fish.

BREADS AND MUFFINS

Biscuits

1¼ cups (100 g.) oatmeal flour
1¼ cups (100 g.) oatmeal
5 tbsp. MCFA oil
½ cup (42 g.) oat bran
2½ tsp. baking powder
¾ cup water
substitute salt (optional)

Preheat oven at 475 degrees. Mix together oatmeal flour, oatmeal, oat bran, baking powder, and substitute salt. Add MCFA oil. Stir with fork until moist and crumbly. Add water and mix well until dough pulls away from bowl. Turn out onto lightly floured surface and knead 30 seconds. Roll dough out ¾ inch thick and use biscuit pattern or medium-sized glass to cut out. Biscuits should be placed on a baking sheet lightly sprayed with a non-stick spray. Reduce heat to 350 degrees and bake 10–12 minutes.

Nutritional value of entire recipe: 1,560 calories, 36.8 g. protein, 18.8 g. fat, 169.4 g. carbohydrate, 4 mg. sodium, and 879 g. potassium.

Oat Bran Crackers

½ cup boiling water
2 tbsp. MCFA oil
1¼ cups (100 g.) oat bran

Preheat oven to 350 degrees. Pour boiling water over MCFA oil and oat bran. Mix well with fork. Shape dough into small 1 oz. balls and press flat into a flat cracker on a cookie sheet lightly sprayed with non-stick spray, making it as flat and thin as you can. Bake 25 to 30 minutes or until light brown. Yield around 8 crackers.

Nutritional value of entire recipe: 552 calories, 15 g. protein, 6 g. fat, 54 g. carbohydrate, 0 mg. sodium, and 360 g. potassium.

Oat Tortillas

½ cup (42 g.) oatmeal flour
½ cup (42 g.) oat bran
5 (150 g.) egg whites
1 cup water
2 tbsp. MCFA oil

Mix all ingredients together until well blended. Batter will appear thin. Heat 7 or 8-inch non-stick skillet and pour small amount of batter in middle of skillet. Shake slightly to spread batter. When tiny bubbles appear on top, pick up edge with spatula and check for doneness. When light brown, turn over and press down with spatula until tortilla appears dry and not wet. Takes about 2 minutes on each side. Makes 6–8 tortillas, depending on size of skillet.

Nutritional value of entire recipe: 692 calories, 32.4 g. protein, 7.2 g. fat, 69.5 g. carbohydrate, 220 mg. sodium, and 565 g. potassium.

Skillet-Cake Bread

1¼ cups (100 g.) oatmeal flour
7 (200 g.) egg whites
1½ tbsp. imitation vanilla butter and nut extract
2 tsp. vanilla
1 tsp. cinnamon
1 tsp. lemon extract
½ tsp. baking soda
1 tsp. baking powder
1 tbsp. MCFA oil

Mix all ingredients in medium-sized bowl with wire whip. Pour batter into hot 12-inch non-stick skillet and shake immediately so that batter covers bottom of skillet. Cook until bubbles form on top and cake seems easy to lift with spatula and turn. Cook one more minute and then remove from skillet and put on round platter. Cut the cake into 4 wedges.

Nutritional value of entire recipe: 606 calories, 36 g. protein, 9 g. fat, 68.2 g. carbohydrate, 294 mg. sodium, and 630 g. potassium.

Sweet Potato–Oat Bran Muffins

1½ (350 g.) grated raw sweet potatoes
2⅔ cups (250 g.) oat bran
1 tbsp. baking powder
1½ tsp. cinnamon
½ tsp. allspice
1¼ cup water
7 (200 g.) egg whites
2 tbsp. MCFA oil

Scrub, peel, and grate sweet potatoes or put through food processor. Place in mixing bowl and add oat bran, baking powder, cinnamon, and allspice. Mix well. Add water and MCFA oil to batter. Beat egg whites and fold into batter. Fill muffin pans sprayed lightly with a non-stick spray. Bake at 325–350 degrees for 20–25 minutes or until a toothpick inserted comes out clean. These muffins can be frozen and reheated in the microwave for 45–60 seconds.

Nutritional value of entire recipe: 1,694 calories, 72.2 g. protein, 18.9 g. fat, 254.1 g. carbohydrate, 328 mg. sodium, and 2,028 g. potassium.

SNACKS

Corn Chips

½ cup boiling water
2 tbsp. MCFA oil
1½ cups (125 g.) corn meal
chili powder to taste (no more than ¼ tsp. recommended unless you really like them hot!)
popcorn salt

Preheat oven to 350 degrees. Pour water over MCFA oil, corn meal, and chili powder. Mix well with fork until dough balls itself together. Shape into small ¾- to 1-inch balls and place far enough apart on non-stick cookie sheet so that they do not touch when pressed flat. Press balls as flat and thin as you can, shaping them however you want (triangles, oval, rectangles, etc.). Sprinkle lightly with pinches of popcorn salt and bake about 30 minutes until edges just start to brown. Chips should be thin and crisp but firm so that they can be used to scoop Mexican Bean Dip or any other you may want to try.

Variations: add 1 tsp. jalapeño juice or other spices to give your chips some zip.

Nutritional value of entire recipe: 672 calories, 11.5 g. protein, 4.7 g. fat, 92.1 g. carbohydrate, 1 mg. sodium, and 355 g. potassium.

Popcorn

½ cup (100 g.) popcorn kernels
3 tbsp. MCFA oil
popcorn salt to taste

In three-quart saucepan, pour popcorn and MCFA oil. Keep heat medium low so that MCFA oil does not scorch. When kernels begin to bubble, start shaking pan over heat until popping slows to just a few seconds in between. Sprinkle with pinches of popcorn salt to taste or add other flavorings. Makes about 5 cups.

Nutritional value of entire recipe: 704 calories, 11.9 g. protein, 4.7 g. fat, 72.1 g. carbohydrate, 3 mg. sodium, and 0 g. potassium.

Potato Chips

1 large (300 g.) potato, with or without skin, depending on your taste

1 tbsp. MCFA oil
pinch of garlic powder
popcorn salt to taste

Slice potatoes very thin, and soak for 15 minutes in MCFA oil and garlic powder. Preheat oven to 325 degrees. Spread potato slices out on non-stick 14″ × 10″ baking sheet, being careful to not overlap them too much, so that they can cook through. Sprinkle with pinches of popcorn salt and bake for about 30 minutes until edges and smaller pieces are brown. Remove from cookie sheet and drain on paper towel if, you wish.

Hint: You can make a bigger batch of chips if you prefer. One 14″ × 10″ sheet holds 300 g. potatoes laid out flat. Also, you can flavor your potato chips with barbecue seasoning powder sprinkled on top, onion powder or finely chopped chives, or even Ranch-flavored party dip mix.

Nutritional value of entire recipe: 342 calories, 6.3 g. protein, .3 g. fat, 51.3 g. carbohydrate, 9 mg. sodium, and 1,221 g. potassium.

DESSERTS

Mock Pumpkin Pudding

(Made with sweet potatoes)
2 (approximately 400 g.) cooked and mashed sweet potatoes
3 (100 g.) egg whites
¼ cup boiling water

1¼ oz. pkg. of unflavored gelatin
1 tsp. pumpkin pie spice
1 tbsp. MCFA oil

Pour water in blender and turn on low. Add gelatin, egg whites, sweet potato, MCFA oil, and pumpkin spice. Blend until mixture has a smooth consistency. Pour into sherbet or dessert glasses and chill until pudding is firm. Top with Whipped Cream. Makes 4 servings.

Nutritional value of entire recipe: 646 calories, 84.9 g. protein, 1.6 g. fat, 106 g. carbohydrate, 216 mg. sodium, and 1,111 g. potassium.

Sweet Potato-Oatmeal Refrigerator Cookies

1¼ cups (100 g.) oatmeal
1 (250 g.) sweet potato
2 tbsp. MCFA oil
1 oz. powdered carbohydrate supplement
2 tsp. cinnamon
2 tsp. vanilla
1 tbsp. water

Mix all ingredients in medium-sized bowl until dough is tacky and can be formed into balls with hands. Roll dough into 1-inch balls and place on platter. Cover and refrigerate at least 1 hour, but overnight is better!

Nutritional value of entire recipe: 951 calories, 21.6 g. protein, 8.2 g. fat, 142.8 g. carbohydrate, 86 mg. sodium, and 1,010 g. potassium.

Appendix C: Nutrition Diary

Date _____   Weight _____

Time	Food and Quantity	Calories	Protein (Grams)	Fat (Grams)	Carbs (Grams)	NA (mg)	K (mg)
Totals							

About the Authors

Nutrition and training expert JOHN PAR-RILLO has been described by a leading bodybuilding magazine as "an exercise and nutrition genius who knows more about maximizing muscle growth and losing body fat than anyone else in the world." Together, his nutrition, supplementation, fascial stretching, training techniques, and body composition charting make up a new—and revolutionary—bodybuilding program.

A former powerlifter and bodybuilder, John has worked with professional and amateur bodybuilders, powerlifters, endurance athletes, pro wrestlers, and other athletes for 20 years, teaching them how to diet and train for maximum performance and results.

John is the author of several manuals on his programs. In addition, he writes nutrition and training articles for various magazines and is a columnist for *Muscle-Mag International, Muscle Training Illustrated,* and *American Fitness Quarterly.*

MAGGIE GREENWOOD-ROBINSON is the coauthor of *BUILT! The New Bodybuilding for Everyone* (with Robert Kennedy) and *Lean Bodies* (with Cliff Sheats).* She is a regular columnist for *Female Bodybuilding,* and her articles have appeared in *Women's Sports and Fitness, Working Woman, Muscle and Fitness, MuscleMag International,* and many other publications.

BUILD BIGGER MUSCLES AND A STRONGER, HEALTHIER BODY WITH BOOKS BY AMERICA'S LEADING AUTHORITIES ON FITNESS AND BODYBUILDING

These books are available at your bookstore or wherever books are sold, or, for your convenience, we'll send them directly to you. Just call 1-800-631-8571 (press 1 for inquiries and orders), or fill out the coupon below and send it to:

**The Putnam Publishing Group
390 Murray Hill Parkway, Dept. B
East Rutherford, NJ 07073**

		Price	
		U.S.	Canada
by Ellington Darden			
_____ Bigger Muscles in 42 Days	399-51706-5	$14.95	$19.50
_____ Big	399-51630-1	14.95	19.50
_____ New High-Intensity Bodybuilding	399-51614-X	15.95	20.95
_____ Super High-Intensity Bodybuilding	399-51220-9	13.95	18.50
_____ 100 High-Intensity Ways to Improve Your Bodybuilding	399-51514-3	14.95	19.50
_____ High-Intensity Strength Training	399-51770-7	15.95	20.95
_____ Big Arms in Six Weeks	399-51432-5	11.95	15.75
_____ Massive Muscles in 10 Weeks	399-51340-X	14.95	19.50
by Robert Kennedy			
_____ Built!	399-51682-4	14.95	19.50
_____ Cuts!	399-51477-5	14.95	19.50
by John Parrillo			
_____ High-Performance Bodybuilding	399-51771-5	15.95	20.95

Subtotal	$	_____
Postage & handling*	$	_____
Sales tax (CA, NJ, NY, PA)	$	_____
Total amount due	$	_____

Payable in U.S. funds (no cash orders accepted). $15.00 minimum for credit card orders.

*Postage & handling: $2.50 for 1 book, 75¢ for each additional book up to a maximum of $6.25.

Enclosed is my ☐ check ☐ money order

Please charge my ☐ Visa   ☐ MasterCard   ☐ American Express

Card #_____ **Expiration date** _____

Signature as on charge card _____

Name _____

Address _____

City _____ **State** _____ **Zip** _____

Please allow six weeks for delivery. Prices subject to change without notice.
Source key #35